THE COMPLETE ANTI-INFLAMMATORY DIET

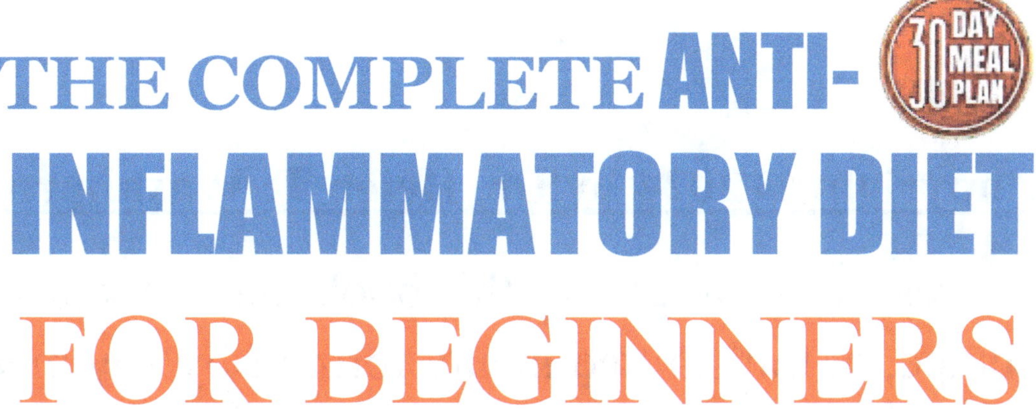

FOR BEGINNERS

Transform Your Health with Stress-Free, Easy and Delicious Recipes to Fight Inflammation and Boost Vitality

Dr. Helen T. Washburn

TABLE OF CONTENTS

The Complete Anti-Inflammatory Diet for Beginners is a recommendation for anyone who wishes to follow a healthy lifestyle. Whether you are making the switch to an anti-inflammatory diet for health reasons, weight loss, or chronic disease prevention, this quick book introduction will provide you with the recipes and information you need to get started.

Your meal plan determines your body's ability to thrive and live a healthy life. You can choose to live a life full of fatigue, restlessness, and chronic diseases, or a life of vibrancy, creativity, and longevity. Your diet significantly impacts your health. The Complete Anti-Inflammatory Diet for Beginners is a book that will guide your choice of diet and enable you to live your life to the fullest. The book gives you an in-depth education on the kinds of meals that you need to start eating to maintain a healthy body. The Complete Anti-Inflammatory Diet for Beginners contains dozens of easy-to-follow recipes to guide your eating habits as you learn about the anti-inflammatory diet. By the end of this book, you will have a comprehensive understanding of the anti-inflammatory diet and the value this brings to your overall health.

Understanding Inflammation and Diet

Inflammation is your body's protective response to injury and stimuli. The immune system sends specialized white blood cells to the injured area to restore the affected tissues to their healthy, functional state. Inflammation can be helpful or harmful. Short-term (acute) inflammation starts quickly and is important in fighting illness and injury. Long-term (chronic) inflammation occurs over a longer period. It is part of the disease process that causes signs of illness. Inflammation is linked to the overactivity of the immune system. Diet clearly plays a role in classic inflammatory diseases, such as rheumatoid arthritis. There's no doubt it is very important in inflammation and obesity. Obesity is now seen as a low-grade inflammatory disease. It's linked to an upregulation of macrophages in adipose tissue (fat tissue). These macrophages drive chronic inflammation in the body.

Maintaining a healthy diet is crucial for reducing inflammation and associated health conditions, such as type-2 diabetes, rheumatoid arthritis, and other autoimmune diseases. Numerous studies have shown that the diet significantly affects the risk of chronic inflammation and disease activity. Some people with certain diseases or conditions may benefit from following an anti-inflammatory diet. It mainly focuses on freshly prepared foods while limiting processed and ultra-processed foods. These mainly include whole grains, fruits, vegetables, plant-based proteins (nuts, beans, seeds, tofu), and anti-inflammatory fats (olive oil, nuts, avocado). Fish and seafood may also be included. Limitations are placed on added sugars, sodium, and low-nutrient snacks and beverages. Avoiding artificial additives, preservatives, and colorings is also recommended. If you are struggling with inflammation or want to maintain better health, consider adopting a healthier diet.

Benefits of an Anti-Inflammatory Diet

Adopting an anti-inflammatory diet can have numerous benefits for your overall health and well-being, including:

- ❖ **Reduced Risk of Chronic Diseases**: By lowering inflammation, you reduce your risk of developing chronic diseases such as heart disease, diabetes, and certain types of cancer.
- ❖ **Improved Digestion**: Anti-inflammatory foods can promote a healthy gut, aiding in better digestion and nutrient absorption.
- ❖ **Enhanced Mental Health**: Some anti-inflammatory foods have been linked to improved mood and cognitive function.
- ❖ **Better Joint Health**: Reducing inflammation can help alleviate symptoms of arthritis and other joint-related issues.
- ❖ **Weight Management**: Many anti-inflammatory foods are nutrient-dense and can help you maintain a healthy weight.
- ❖ **Boosted Immune System:** An anti-inflammatory diet can strengthen your immune system, making it easier for your body to fight off infections and illnesses.
- ❖ **Increased Energy Levels:** Eating a balanced diet that includes anti-inflammatory foods can help maintain steady energy levels throughout the day.
- ❖ **Enhanced Skin Health:** Chronic inflammation can lead to various skin issues, including acne, eczema, and premature aging. An anti-inflammatory diet, rich in antioxidants and healthy fats, can promote healthier skin by reducing inflammation and supporting skin repair and regeneration.
- ❖ **Reduced Inflammation Markers:** Studies have shown that an anti-inflammatory diet can reduce markers of inflammation in the body, such as C-reactive protein (CRP) and interleukin-6 (IL-6). Lowering these markers can indicate a reduction in overall inflammation, which is beneficial for long-term health and disease prevention.

Essential Ingredients and Pantry Staples

To successfully follow an anti-inflammatory diet, stocking your pantry with the right ingredients is crucial. Here are some essential staples:

- ❖ **Fruits and Vegetables**: Aim for a variety of colorful fruits and vegetables, such as berries, leafy greens, tomatoes, and bell peppers.
- ❖ **Healthy Fats**: Add foods like nuts, seeds, olive oil, and avocados that are high in healthy fats.
- ❖ **Whole Grains**: Go for whole grains such as quinoa, brown rice, and oats instead of refined grains.
- ❖ **Lean Proteins**: Choose lean protein sources like chicken, turkey, fish, and plant-based proteins such as beans and lentils.
- ❖ **Herbs and Spices**: Use anti-inflammatory spices like turmeric, ginger, garlic, and cinnamon to add flavor to your dishes.
- ❖ **Healthy Beverages**: Drink green tea, herbal teas, and plenty of water. Avoid sugary drinks and limit alcohol consumption.

Essential Tools and Accessories

Having the right tools and accessories can make preparation of anti-inflammatory meals easier and more enjoyable. Here are items you may find helpful:

- **High-Quality Knife Set**: Sharp knives make chopping fruits, vegetables, and proteins much easier and safer.
- **Cutting Boards**: Have multiple cutting boards to avoid cross-contamination between raw meats and fresh produce.
- **Blender or Food Processor**: Ideal for making smoothies, soups, and sauces.
- **Spice Grinder**: Freshly ground spices can enhance the flavor and anti-inflammatory properties of your dishes.
- **Storage Containers**: Keep prepped ingredients and leftovers fresh with a variety of storage containers.
- **Non-Stick Cookware**: Reduces the need for excess oils and makes for easy cleanup.
- **Measuring Cups and Spoons**: Essential for following recipes accurately.
- **Mixing Bowls:** A set of mixing bowls in various sizes is useful for mixing ingredients, marinating, and even serving.
- **Vegetable Peeler:** A good vegetable peeler makes peeling fruits and vegetables quick and easy.
- **Steamer Basket:** A steamer basket is perfect for steaming vegetables, which helps retain their nutrients.
- **Baking Sheets and Pans:** Non-stick or silicone baking sheets and pans are great for roasting vegetables, baking fish, and making healthy snacks.
- **Salad Spinner:** A salad spinner is essential for thoroughly washing and drying leafy greens.
- **Mandoline Slicer:** A mandoline slicer allows you to slice vegetables uniformly and quickly.
- **Immersion Blender:** An immersion blender, also known as a hand blender, is useful for pureeing soups directly in the pot, blending smoothies, and making dressings.
- **Air Fryer:** An air fryer allows you to cook foods with little to no oil while achieving a crispy texture.

Meal Planning and Preparation Tips

Planning and preparing your meals in advance can make it easier to stick to an anti-inflammatory diet. Here are some tips to help you get started:

- **Plan Your Meals**: Make a weekly menu that consists of a range of foods that reduce inflammation. This helps ensure you get a balanced intake of nutrients.
- **Prep Ingredients in Advance**: Chop vegetables, cook grains, and prepare proteins in advance to save time during the week.
- **Batch Cooking**: Cook larger portions of meals and store them in the refrigerator or freezer for easy access during busy days.

❖ **Healthy Snacks**: Keep healthy snacks like cut-up veggies, hummus, and nuts on hand to avoid reaching for inflammatory options.

❖ **Stay Hydrated**: Drinking plenty of water is essential for reducing inflammation and maintaining overall health.

❖ **Use Leftovers Wisely:** Repurpose leftovers to create new meals.

❖ **Invest in Quality Storage Containers:** Having a variety of storage containers in different sizes will help you keep your prepped ingredients and meals fresh.

❖ **Keep a Well-Stocked Pantry:** A well-stocked pantry makes it easier to whip up anti-inflammatory meals without frequent trips to the grocery store.

❖ **Experiment with New Recipes:** Variety is key to a sustainable diet. To keep your meals engaging and fun, try out different recipes and components.

❖ **Make It a Family Affair:** Involve your family in organizing and preparing meals. This can be a fun and educational activity that helps everyone understand the importance of healthy eating.

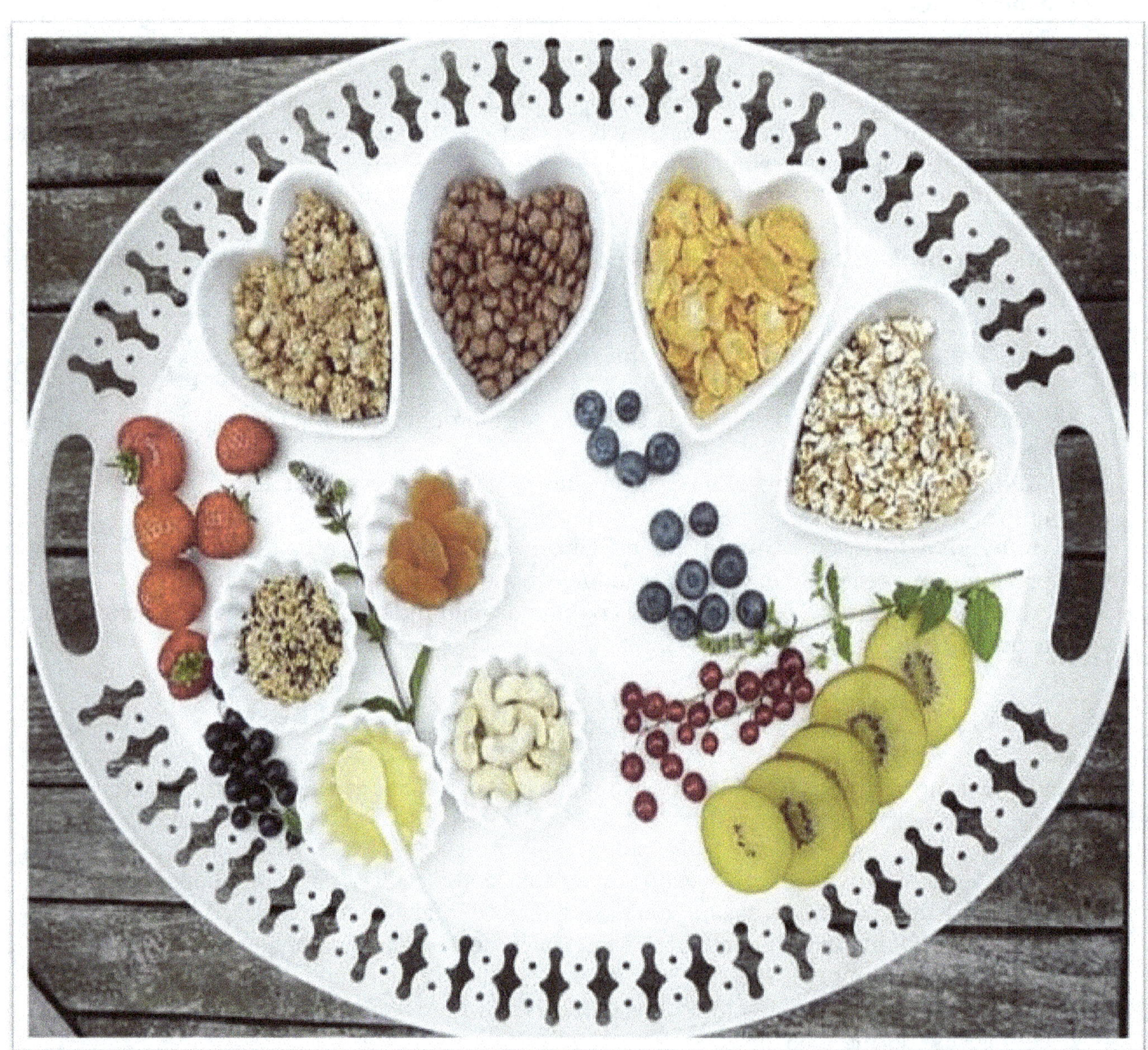

Turmeric and Ginger Smoothie

Prep Time: 10 minutes | Cooking Time: 0 minutes | Servings: 2

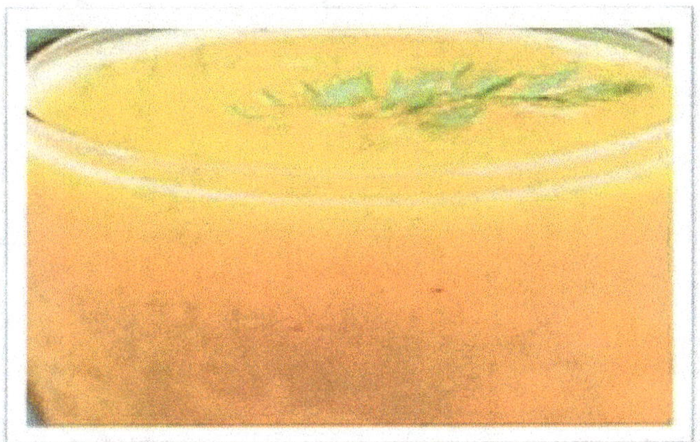

Ingredients:

- 1 cup unsweetened almond milk
- 1 banana
- 1/2 cup frozen mango chunks
- 1/2 cup frozen pineapple chunks
- 1 teaspoon ground turmeric
- 1/2 teaspoon ground ginger
- 1 tablespoon chia seeds
- 1 teaspoon honey (optional)

Instructions:

1. Add the almond milk, banana, mango, pineapple, turmeric, ginger, and chia seeds to a blender.
2. Blend on high until smooth and creamy.
3. Taste and add honey if desired for extra sweetness.
4. Pour into two glasses and serve immediately.

Nutritional Information: Calories: 150 | Protein: 3g | Carbohydrates: 34g | Fat: 3g | Fiber: 6g | Sugar: 20g

Overnight Oats with Chia Seeds

Prep Time: 10 minutes | Cooking Time: 0 minutes | Servings: 2

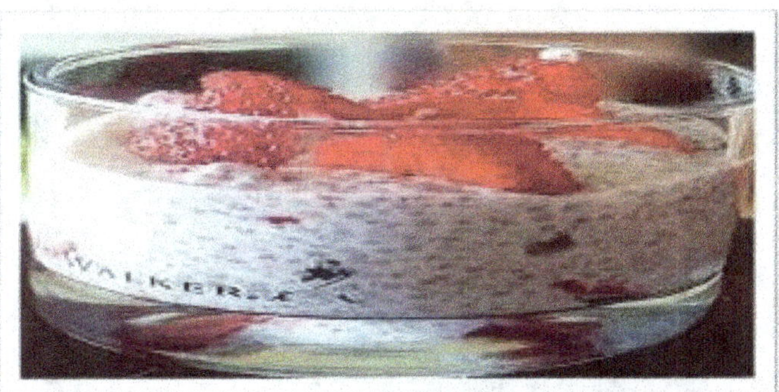

Ingredients:

- 1 cup rolled oats
- 1 cup unsweetened almond milk
- 1/2 cup Greek yogurt
- 2 tablespoons chia seeds
- 1 tablespoon honey
- 1 teaspoon vanilla extract
- 1/2 cup fresh berries (blueberries, strawberries, or raspberries)

Instructions:

1. In a medium-sized bowl, combine rolled oats, almond milk, Greek yogurt, chia seeds, honey, and vanilla extract.
2. Stir well to combine all ingredients.
3. Divide the mixture into two mason jars or airtight containers.
4. Top each jar with fresh berries.
5. Cover and refrigerate overnight.
6. In the morning, stir the oats and enjoy cold or warm them up if preferred.

Nutritional Information: Calories: 250 | Protein: 10g | Carbohydrates: 40g | Fat: 6g | Fiber: 8g | Sugar: 15g

Anti-Inflammatory Green Juice

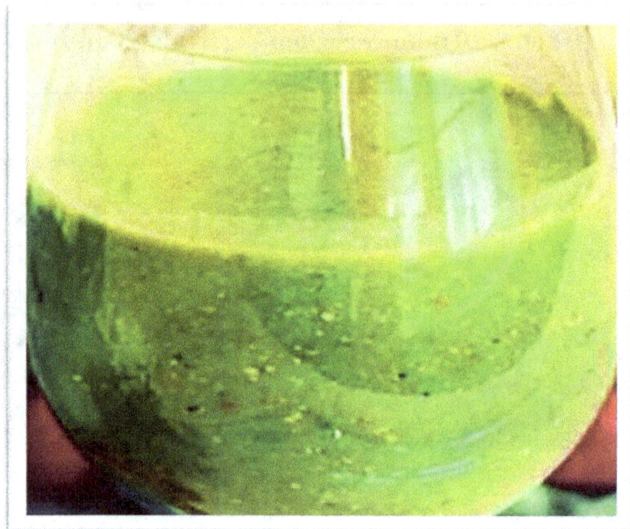

Ingredients:

- 2 cups spinach
- 1 cucumber, peeled and chopped
- 2 green apples, cored and chopped
- 1-inch piece of ginger, peeled
- 1/2 lemon, juiced
- 1 cup coconut water

Instructions:

1. Add spinach, cucumber, green apples, ginger, lemon juice, and coconut water to a blender.
2. Blend on high until smooth.
3. Strain the juice through a fine mesh sieve or cheesecloth into a pitcher.
4. Pour into two glasses and serve immediately.

Nutritional Information: Calories: 90 | Protein: 2g | Carbohydrates: 22g | Fat: 0g | Fiber: 4g | Sugar: 15g

Quinoa Breakfast Bowl with Berries

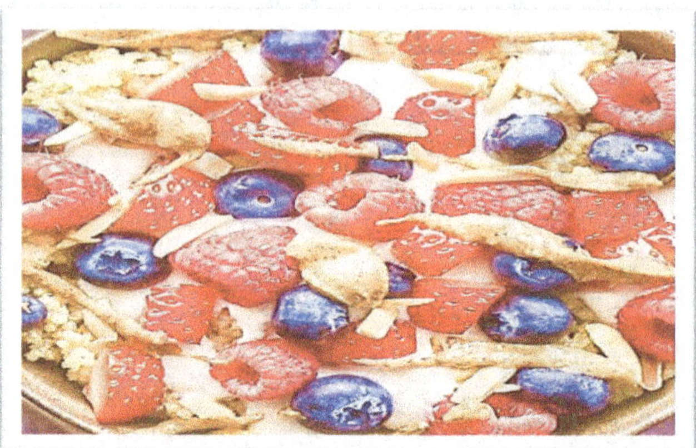

Ingredients:

- 1/2 cup quinoa, rinsed
- 1 cup water
- 1/2 cup almond milk
- 1 tablespoon honey
- 1 teaspoon vanilla extract
- 1/2 cup fresh berries (blueberries, strawberries, or raspberries)
- 1 tablespoon chopped nuts (almonds, walnuts, or pecans)

Instructions:

1. In a medium saucepan, combine quinoa and water. Bring to a boil over medium heat.
2. Reduce heat to low, cover, and simmer for 15 minutes, or until quinoa is cooked and water is absorbed.
3. Remove from heat and stir in almond milk, honey, and vanilla extract.
4. Divide quinoa mixture into two bowls.
5. Top with fresh berries and chopped nuts.
6. Serve warm.

Nutritional Information: Calories: 220 | Protein: 7g | Carbohydrates: 38g | Fat: 5g | Fiber: 6g | Sugar: 12g

Avocado and Spinach Smoothie

Prep Time: 10 minutes | Cooking Time: 0 minutes | Servings: 2

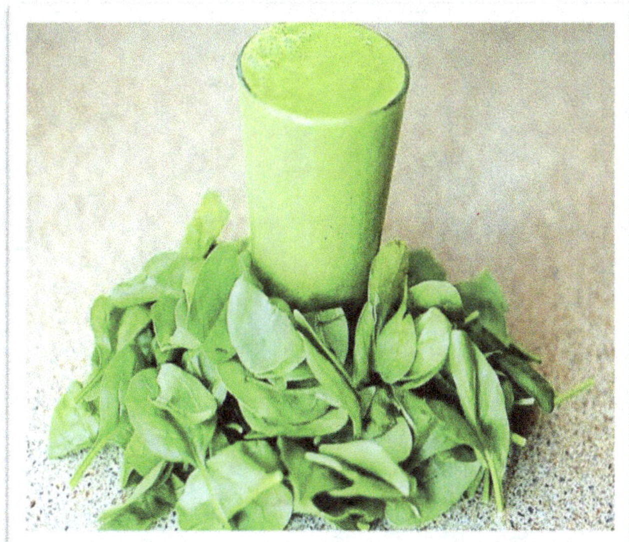

Ingredients:

- 1 ripe avocado
- 2 cups fresh spinach
- 1 banana
- 1 cup unsweetened almond milk
- 1 tablespoon chia seeds
- 1 teaspoon honey (optional)

Instructions:

1. Cut the avocado in half, remove the pit, and scoop the flesh into a blender.
2. Add the spinach, banana, almond milk, chia seeds, and honey (if using).
3. Blend on high until smooth and creamy.
4. Pour into two glasses and serve immediately.

Nutritional Information: Calories: 200 | Protein: 4g | Carbohydrates: 26g | Fat: 10g | Fiber: 8g | Sugar: 12g

Sweet Potato and Black Bean Breakfast Hash

Prep Time: 15 minutes | Cooking Time: 25 minutes | Servings: 2

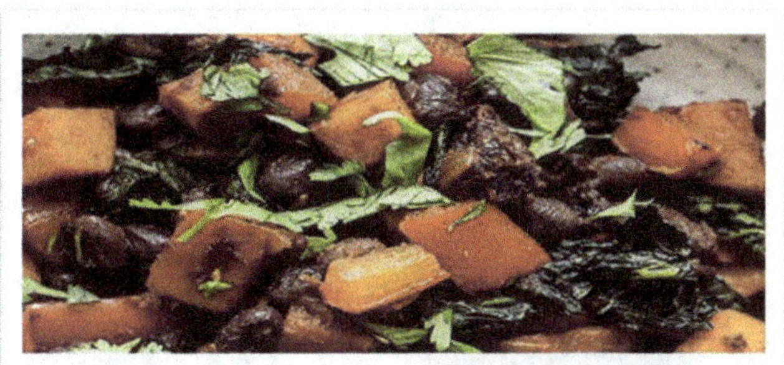

Ingredients:

- 1 large sweet potato, peeled and diced
- 1 tablespoon olive oil
- 1/2 onion, diced
- 1 bell pepper, diced
- 1 can (15 oz) black beans, drained and rinsed
- 1 teaspoon ground cumin
- 1/2 teaspoon smoked paprika
- Salt and pepper to taste
- 2 tablespoons fresh cilantro, chopped

Instructions:

1. Preheat oven to 400°F (200°C).
2. Toss the diced sweet potato with olive oil, salt, and pepper.
3. Spread sweet potato on a baking sheet and roast for 20 minutes, or until tender.
4. In a large skillet, heat a bit of olive oil over medium heat.
5. Add onion and bell pepper, sauté until softened, about 5 minutes.
6. Add roasted sweet potato, black beans, cumin, and smoked paprika to the skillet. Stir to combine.
7. Cook for an additional 5 minutes, stirring occasionally, until everything is heated through.
8. Sprinkle with fresh cilantro before serving.

Nutritional Information: Calories: 320 | Protein: 10g | Carbohydrates: 55g | Fat: 8g | Fiber: 14g | Sugar: 8g

Chia Seed Pudding with Berries

Prep Time: 10 minutes | Cooking Time: 0 minutes | Servings: 2

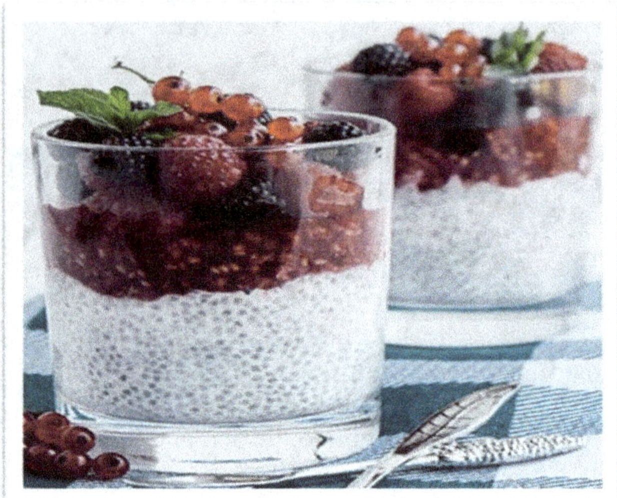

Ingredients:

- 1/4 cup chia seeds
- 1 cup unsweetened almond milk
- 1 tablespoon honey
- 1/2 teaspoon vanilla extract
- 1/2 cup fresh berries (blueberries, strawberries, or raspberries)

Instructions:

1. In a medium bowl, combine chia seeds, almond milk, honey, and vanilla extract.
2. Stir well to combine.
3. Cover and refrigerate for at least 4 hours or overnight.
4. Stir the pudding to break up any clumps before serving.
5. Divide into two bowls and top with fresh berries.

Nutritional Information: Calories: 200 | Protein: 5g | Carbohydrates: 28g | Fat: 8g | Fiber: 10g | Sugar: 14g

Spinach and Mushroom Frittata

Prep Time: 10 minutes | Cooking Time: 20 minutes | Servings: 4

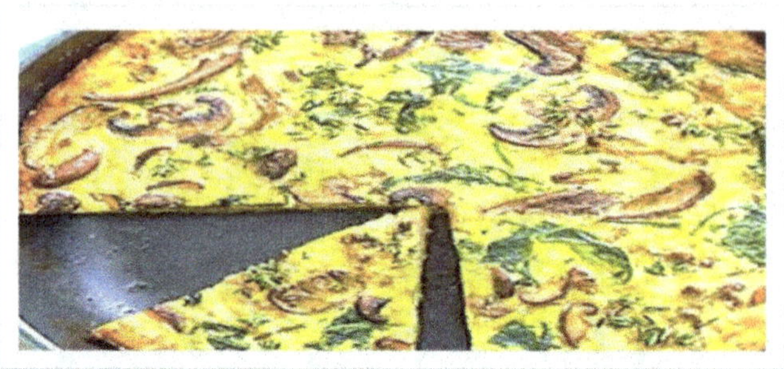

Ingredients:

- 1 tablespoon olive oil
- 1/2 onion, diced
- 1 cup mushrooms, sliced
- 2 cups fresh spinach
- 6 large eggs
- 1/4 cup milk (dairy or non-dairy)
- Salt and pepper to taste
- 1/4 cup feta cheese, crumbled (optional)

Instructions:

1. Preheat the oven to 350°F (175°C).
2. In a large oven-safe skillet, heat olive oil over medium heat.
3. Add onion and mushrooms, sauté until softened, about 5 minutes.
4. Add spinach and cook until wilted, about 2 minutes.
5. In a medium bowl, whisk together eggs, milk, salt, and pepper.
6. Pour egg mixture into the skillet over the vegetables.
7. Cook on the stove for about 5 minutes, until the edges start to set.
8. Transfer the skillet to the oven and bake for 10-15 minutes, or until the frittata is fully set.
9. Remove from the oven and let cool slightly before slicing.
10. Sprinkle with feta cheese, if desired, before serving.

Nutritional Information: Calories: 180 | Protein: 12g | Carbohydrates: 5g | Fat: 13g | Fiber: 2g | Sugar: 2g

Hummus and Veggie Platter

Prep Time: 15 minutes | Cooking Time: 0 minutes | Servings: 4

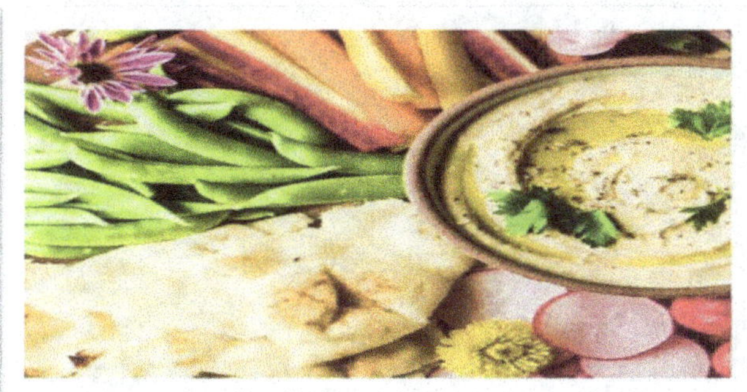

Ingredients:

- 1 can (15 oz) chickpeas, drained and rinsed
- 1/4 cup tahini
- 2 tablespoons olive oil
- 2 cloves garlic
- Juice of 1 lemon
- 1/2 teaspoon ground cumin
- Salt to taste
- Assorted fresh vegetables (carrots, celery, bell peppers, cucumbers), cut into sticks

Instructions:

1. In a food processor, combine chickpeas, tahini, olive oil, garlic, lemon juice, cumin, and salt.
2. Blend until smooth, adding a little water if necessary to achieve desired consistency.
3. Transfer hummus to a serving bowl.
4. Arrange fresh vegetable sticks around the hummus bowl.
5. Serve immediately or refrigerate until ready to serve.

Nutritional Information: Calories: 220 | Protein: 6g | Carbohydrates: 20g | Fat: 12g | Fiber: 6g | Sugar: 3g

Turmeric Roasted Chickpeas

Prep Time: 10 minutes | Cooking Time: 30 minutes | Servings: 4

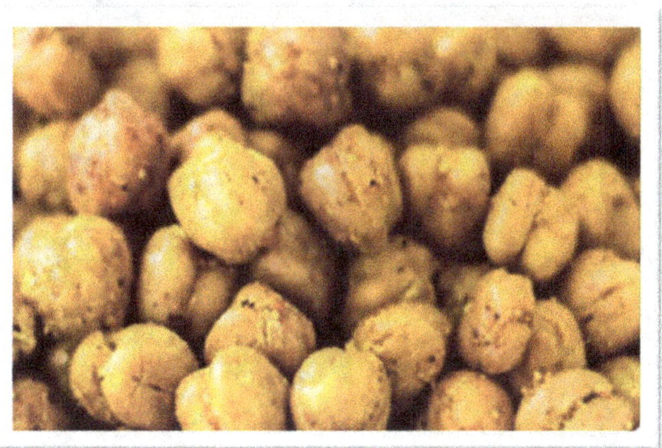

Ingredients:

- 1 can (15 oz) chickpeas, drained and rinsed
- 1 tablespoon olive oil
- 1 teaspoon ground turmeric
- 1/2 teaspoon ground cumin
- 1/2 teaspoon smoked paprika
- 1/4 teaspoon salt

Instructions:

1. Preheat oven to 400°F (200°C).
2. Pat chickpeas dry with a paper towel.
3. In a bowl, toss chickpeas with olive oil, turmeric, cumin, smoked paprika, and salt.
4. Spread chickpeas in a single layer on a baking sheet.
5. Roast for 25-30 minutes, shaking the pan halfway through, until chickpeas are golden and crispy.
6. Let cool slightly before serving.

Nutritional Information: Calories: 140 | Protein: 6g | Carbohydrates: 20g | Fat: 5g | Fiber: 6g | Sugar: 1g

Cucumber and Avocado Bites

Prep Time: 10 minutes | Cooking Time: 0 minutes | Servings: 4

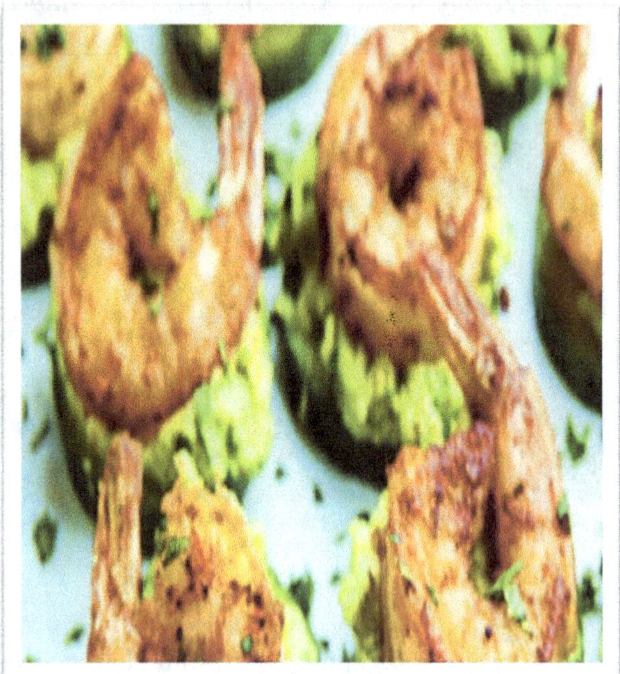

Ingredients:

- 1 large cucumber, sliced into rounds
- 1 ripe avocado, mashed
- Juice of 1/2 lemon
- Salt and pepper to taste
- Fresh dill, for garnish

Instructions:

1. In a small bowl, mash the avocado with lemon juice, salt, and pepper.
2. Place cucumber rounds on a serving platter.
3. Top each cucumber round with a spoonful of mashed avocado.
4. Garnish with fresh dill.
5. Serve immediately.

Nutritional Information: Calories: 80 | Protein: 1g | Carbohydrates: 8g | Fat: 6g | Fiber: 4g | Sugar: 2g

Spicy Kale Chips

Prep Time: 10 minutes | Cooking Time: 20 minutes | Servings: 4

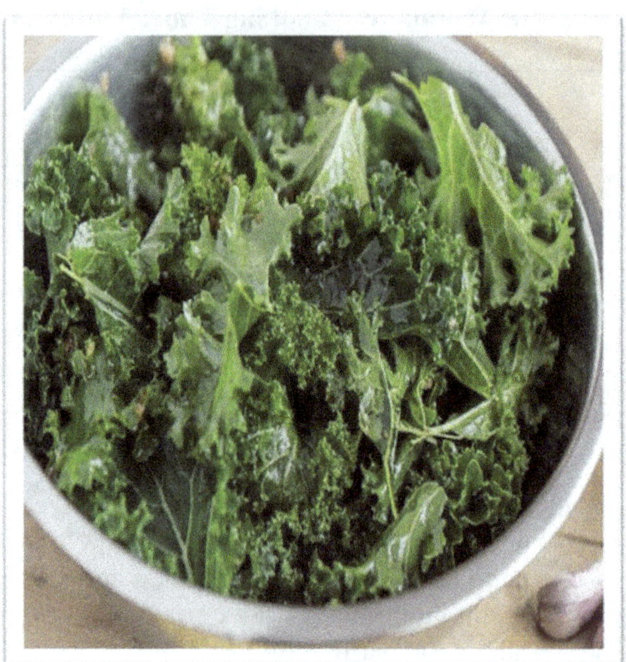

Ingredients:

- 1 bunch kale, washed and torn into bite-sized pieces
- 1 tablespoon olive oil
- 1/2 teaspoon smoked paprika
- 1/4 teaspoon cayenne pepper
- 1/4 teaspoon salt

Instructions:

1. Preheat the oven to 350°F (175°C).
2. In a large bowl, toss kale with olive oil, smoked paprika, cayenne pepper, and salt.
3. Spread kale in a single layer on a baking sheet.
4. Bake for 15-20 minutes, until kale is crispy.
5. Let cool slightly before serving.

Nutritional Information: Calories: 60 | Protein: 2g | Carbohydrates: 7g | Fat: 3g | Fiber: 2g | Sugar: 0g

Almond and Berry Energy Balls

Prep Time: 15 minutes | Cooking Time: 0 minutes | Servings: 4

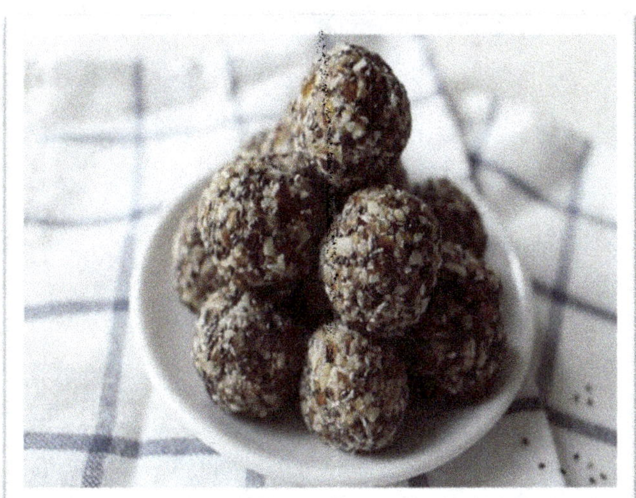

Ingredients:

- 1 cup almonds
- 1 cup mixed dried berries
- 1/4 cup unsweetened shredded coconut
- 2 tablespoons chia seeds
- 1 tablespoon honey
- 1/2 teaspoon vanilla extract

Instructions:

1. In a food processor, pulse almonds until finely ground.
2. Add dried berries, shredded coconut, chia seeds, honey, and vanilla extract.
3. Blend until mixture comes together and forms a dough.
4. Roll the mixture into small balls.
5. Refrigerate for at least 30 minutes before serving.

Nutritional Information: Calories: 180 | Protein: 4g | Carbohydrates: 18g | Fat: 10g | Fiber: 5g | Sugar: 12g

Fresh Vegetable Spring Rolls with Ginger Peanut Sauce

Prep Time: 20 minutes | Cooking Time: 0 minutes | Servings: 4

Ingredients:

- 8 rice paper wrappers
- 1 cup shredded carrots
- 1 cup thinly sliced bell peppers
- 1 cup thinly sliced cucumber
- 1 cup shredded purple cabbage
- 1/2 cup fresh mint leaves
- 1/2 cup fresh cilantro leaves
- 1/2 cup cooked rice noodles (optional)

Ginger Peanut Sauce:

- 1/4 cup peanut butter
- 2 tablespoons soy sauce
- 1 tablespoon rice vinegar
- 1 teaspoon grated ginger
- 1 tablespoon honey
- Water, as needed for thinning

Instructions:

1. Prepare the ginger peanut sauce by whisking together peanut butter, soy sauce, rice vinegar, grated ginger, and honey in a small bowl. Add water as needed to achieve a smooth consistency.
2. Fill a shallow dish with warm water. Dip one rice paper wrapper into the water for about 10 seconds, until pliable.
3. Place the softened wrapper on a clean surface. In the center, layer a small amount of shredded carrots, bell peppers, cucumber, cabbage, mint, cilantro, and rice noodles (if using).
4. Fold the sides of the wrapper over the filling, then roll up tightly from the bottom.
5. Repeat with remaining wrappers and fillings.
6. Serve the spring rolls with the ginger peanut sauce.

Nutritional Information: Calories: 200 | Protein: 5g | Carbohydrates: 30g | Fat: 8g | Fiber: 5g | Sugar: 6g

Baked Zucchini Fries

Prep Time: 15 minutes | Cooking Time: 25 minutes | Servings: 4

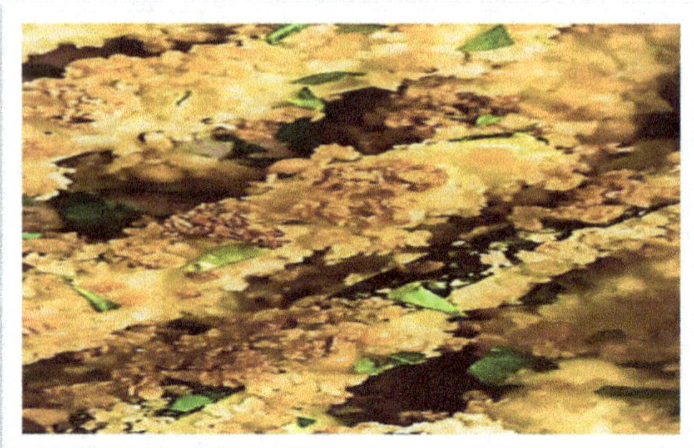

Ingredients:

- 2 large zucchinis, cut into fries
- 1/2 cup almond flour
- 1/4 cup grated Parmesan cheese
- 1 teaspoon garlic powder
- 1 teaspoon paprika
- Salt and pepper to taste
- 1 large egg, beaten

Instructions:

1. Preheat oven to 425°F (220°C). Line a baking sheet with parchment paper.
2. In a shallow bowl, combine almond flour, Parmesan cheese, garlic powder, paprika, salt, and pepper.
3. Dip each zucchini fry into the beaten egg, then coat with the almond flour mixture.
4. Place the coated zucchini fries on the prepared baking sheet.
5. Bake for 20-25 minutes, until golden and crispy.
6. Serve immediately with your favorite dipping sauce.

Nutritional Information: Calories: 120 | Protein: 6g | Carbohydrates: 8g | Fat: 7g | Fiber: 2g | Sugar: 3g

Roasted Red Pepper Hummus

Prep Time: 15 minutes | Cooking Time: 0 minutes | Servings: 4

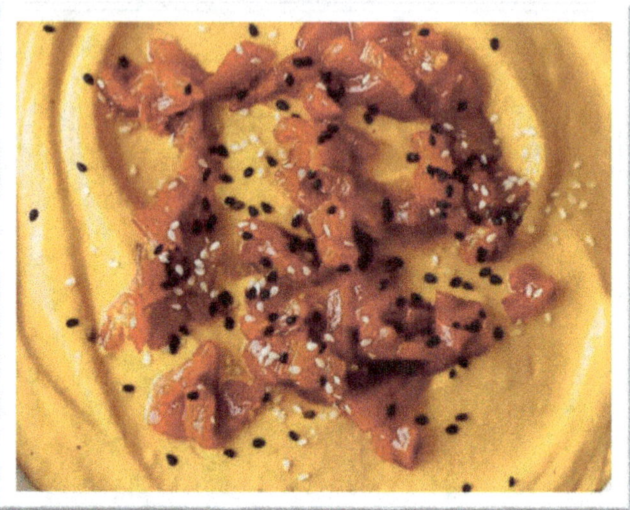

Ingredients:

- 1 can (15 oz) chickpeas, drained and rinsed
- 1/2 cup roasted red peppers
- 1/4 cup tahini
- 2 tablespoons olive oil
- 2 cloves garlic
- Juice of 1 lemon
- 1/2 teaspoon ground cumin
- Salt to taste

Instructions:

1. In a food processor, combine chickpeas, roasted red peppers, tahini, olive oil, garlic, lemon juice, cumin, and salt.
2. Blend until smooth, adding a little water if necessary to achieve desired consistency.
3. Transfer hummus to a serving bowl.
4. Serve with fresh vegetables, pita chips, or as a spread.

Nutritional Information: Calories: 150 | Protein: 5g | Carbohydrates: 16g | Fat: 8g | Fiber: 4g | Sugar: 2g

Golden Turmeric Lentil Soup

Prep Time: 10 minutes | Cooking Time: 30 minutes | Servings: 4

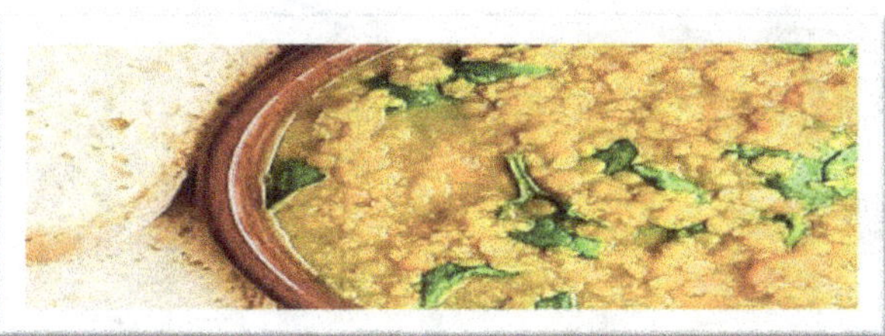

Ingredients:

- 1 tablespoon olive oil
- 1 onion, diced
- 2 cloves garlic, minced
- 1 tablespoon ground turmeric
- 1 teaspoon ground cumin
- 1 teaspoon ground ginger
- 1 cup red lentils, rinsed
- 4 cups vegetable broth
- 1 can (14.5 oz) diced tomatoes
- 1 cup coconut milk
- Salt and pepper to taste
- Fresh cilantro, for garnish

Instructions:

1. In a large pot, heat olive oil over medium heat.
2. Add onion and garlic, sauté until softened, about 5 minutes.
3. Stir in turmeric, cumin, and ginger, cooking for 1 minute until fragrant.
4. Add lentils, vegetable broth, and diced tomatoes. Bring to a boil.
5. Reduce heat, cover, and simmer for 20 minutes, until lentils are tender.
6. Stir in coconut milk, season with salt and pepper.
7. Simmer for an additional 5 minutes.
8. Serve hot, garnished with fresh cilantro.

Nutritional Information: Calories: 250 | Protein: 10g | Carbohydrates: 30g | Fat: 10g | Fiber: 8g | Sugar: 6g

Chicken and Vegetable Broth

Prep Time: 15 minutes | Cooking Time: 1 hour 30 minutes | Servings: 6

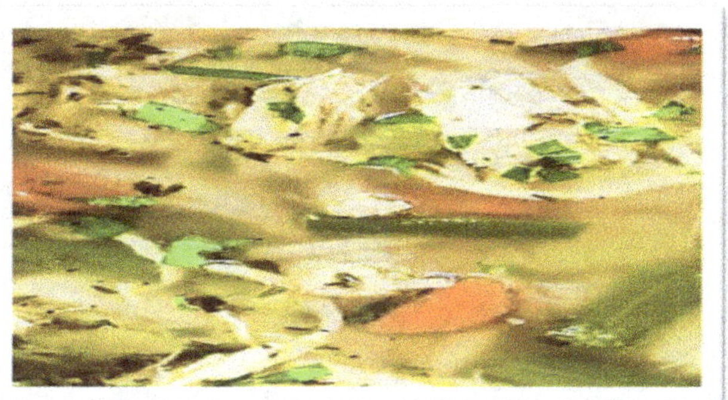

Ingredients:

- 1 whole chicken (about 3-4 pounds), giblets removed
- 8 cups water
- 2 carrots, chopped
- 2 celery stalks, chopped
- 1 onion, quartered
- 3 cloves garlic, smashed
- 1 bay leaf
- 1 teaspoon whole black peppercorns
- Salt to taste
- Fresh parsley, for garnish

Instructions:

1. In a large pot, combine chicken, water, carrots, celery, onion, garlic, bay leaf, and peppercorns.
2. Bring to a boil over medium-high heat.
3. Reduce heat, cover, and simmer for 1.5 hours, skimming any foam that rises to the surface.
4. Remove chicken and vegetables from the pot.
5. Strain the broth through a fine mesh sieve into another pot.
6. Season with salt.
7. Serve hot, garnished with fresh parsley.

Nutritional Information: Calories: 150 | Protein: 20g | Carbohydrates: 5g | Fat: 5g | Fiber: 1g | Sugar: 2g

Sweet Potato and Coconut Soup

Prep Time: 10 minutes | Cooking Time: 30 minutes | Servings: 4

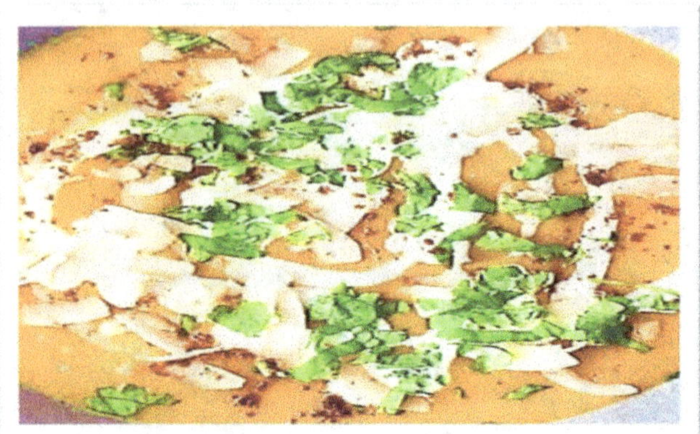

Ingredients:

- 1 tablespoon olive oil
- 1 onion, diced
- 2 cloves garlic, minced
- 1 tablespoon grated ginger
- 3 sweet potatoes, peeled and cubed
- 4 cups vegetable broth
- 1 can (14 oz) coconut milk
- Salt and pepper to taste
- Fresh cilantro, for garnish

Instructions:

1. In a large pot, heat olive oil over medium heat.
2. Add onion, garlic, and ginger, sauté until softened, about 5 minutes.
3. Add sweet potatoes and vegetable broth. Bring to a boil.
4. Reduce heat, cover, and simmer for 20 minutes, until sweet potatoes are tender.
5. Use an immersion blender to puree the soup until smooth.
6. Stir in coconut milk, season with salt and pepper.
7. Simmer for an additional 5 minutes.
8. Serve hot, garnished with fresh cilantro.

Nutritional Information: Calories: 280 | Protein: 4g | Carbohydrates: 40g | Fat: 12g | Fiber: 6g | Sugar: 10g

Miso Soup with Tofu and Seaweed

Prep Time: 10 minutes | Cooking Time: 10 minutes | Servings: 4

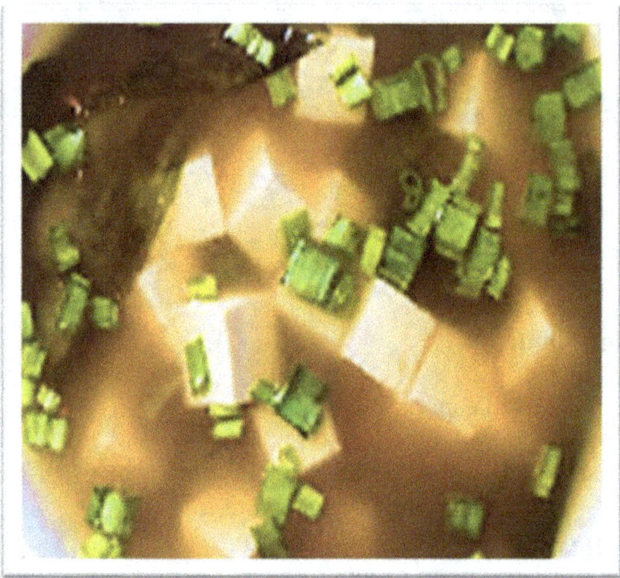

Ingredients:

- 4 cups water
- 3 tablespoons miso paste
- 1/2 cup cubed tofu
- 1/4 cup sliced green onions
- 1/4 cup dried seaweed
- 1 tablespoon soy sauce

Instructions:

1. In a medium pot, bring water to a simmer.
2. Whisk in miso paste until fully dissolved.
3. Add tofu, green onions, and seaweed.
4. Simmer for 5 minutes, until tofu is heated through and seaweed is rehydrated.
5. Stir in soy sauce.
6. Serve hot.

Nutritional Information: Calories: 80 | Protein: 5g | Carbohydrates: 8g | Fat: 3g | Fiber: 2g | Sugar: 2g

Hearty Quinoa and Vegetable Stew

Prep Time: 15 minutes | Cooking Time: 30 minutes | Servings: 4

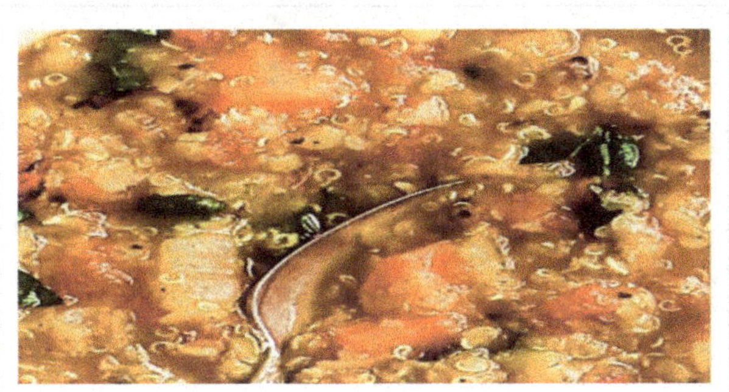

Ingredients:

- 1 tablespoon olive oil
- 1 onion, diced
- 2 cloves garlic, minced
- 2 carrots, chopped
- 2 celery stalks, chopped
- 1 zucchini, chopped
- 1 cup quinoa, rinsed
- 4 cups vegetable broth
- 1 can (14.5 oz) diced tomatoes
- 1 teaspoon dried thyme
- 1 teaspoon dried basil
- Salt and pepper to taste
- Fresh parsley, for garnish

Instructions:

1. In a large pot, heat olive oil over medium heat.
2. Add onion and garlic, sauté until softened, about 5 minutes.
3. Add carrots, celery, and zucchini, cooking for another 5 minutes.
4. Stir in quinoa, vegetable broth, diced tomatoes, thyme, and basil.
5. Bring to a boil, then reduce heat, cover, and simmer for 20 minutes, until quinoa is cooked and vegetables are tender.
6. Season with salt and pepper.
7. Serve hot, garnished with fresh parsley.

Nutritional Information: Calories: 250 | Protein: 8g | Carbohydrates: 42g | Fat: 5g | Fiber: 8g | Sugar: 8g

Butternut Squash and Apple Soup

Prep Time: 15 minutes | Cooking Time: 30 minutes | Servings: 4

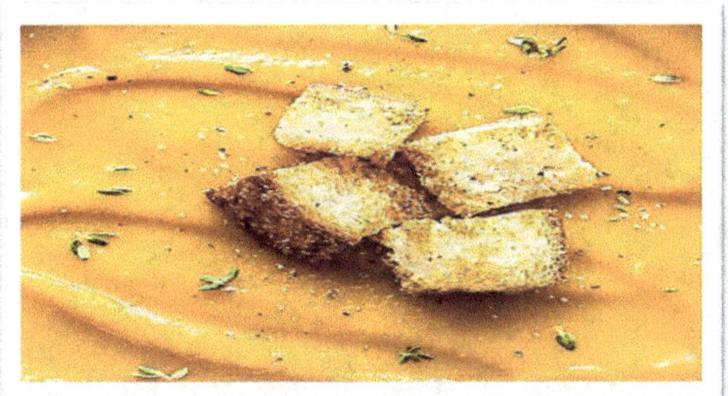

Ingredients:

- 1 tablespoon olive oil
- 1 onion, diced
- 2 cloves garlic, minced
- 1 butternut squash, peeled and cubed
- 2 apples, peeled, cored, and chopped
- 4 cups vegetable broth
- 1 teaspoon ground cinnamon
- Salt and pepper to taste
- Fresh thyme, for garnish

Instructions:

1. In a large pot, heat olive oil over medium heat.
2. Add onion and garlic, sauté until softened, about 5 minutes.
3. Add butternut squash, apples, and vegetable broth. Bring to a boil.
4. Reduce heat, cover, and simmer for 20 minutes, until squash and apples are tender.
5. Use an immersion blender to puree the soup until smooth.
6. Stir in ground cinnamon, season with salt and pepper.
7. Simmer for an additional 5 minutes.
8. Serve hot, garnished with fresh thyme.

Nutritional Information: Calories: 200 | Protein: 2g | Carbohydrates: 45g | Fat: 4g | Fiber: 8g | Sugar: 20g

Tomato Basil Soup with Quinoa

Prep Time: 10 minutes | Cooking Time: 25 minutes | Servings: 4

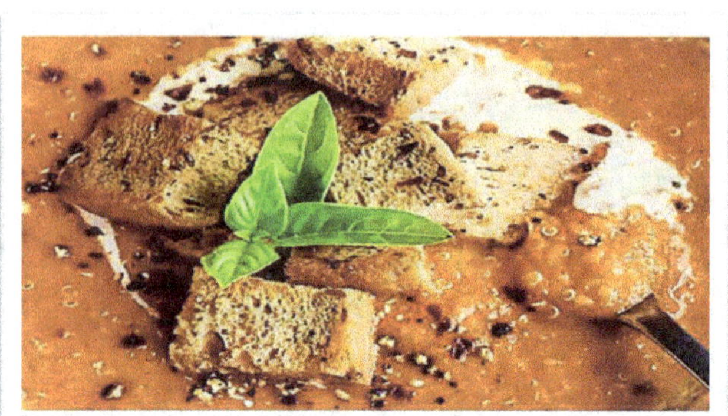

Ingredients:

- 1 tablespoon olive oil
- 1 onion, diced
- 2 cloves garlic, minced
- 1 can (28 oz) crushed tomatoes
- 4 cups vegetable broth
- 1/2 cup quinoa, rinsed
- 1 teaspoon dried basil
- Salt and pepper to taste
- Fresh basil, for garnish

Instructions:

1. In a large pot, heat olive oil over medium heat.
2. Add onion and garlic, sauté until softened, about 5 minutes.
3. Stir in crushed tomatoes, vegetable broth, quinoa, and dried basil.
4. Bring to a boil, then reduce heat, cover, and simmer for 20 minutes, until quinoa is cooked.
5. Season with salt and pepper.
6. Serve hot, garnished with fresh basil.

Nutritional Information: Calories: 180 | Protein: 6g | Carbohydrates: 32g | Fat: 5g | Fiber: 6g | Sugar: 12g

Curried Cauliflower Soup

Prep Time: 10 minutes | Cooking Time: 25 minutes | Servings: 4

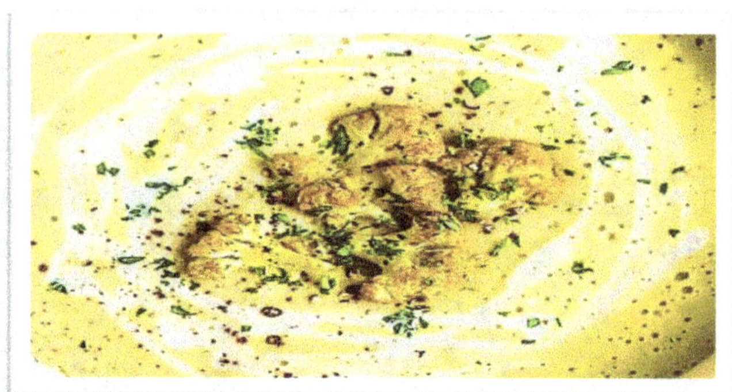

Ingredients:

- 1 tablespoon olive oil
- 1 onion, diced
- 2 cloves garlic, minced
- 1 tablespoon curry powder
- 1 large head cauliflower, chopped
- 4 cups vegetable broth
- 1 can (14.5 oz) coconut milk
- Salt and pepper to taste
- Fresh cilantro, for garnish

Instructions:

1. In a large pot, heat olive oil over medium heat.
2. Add onion and garlic, sauté until softened, about 5 minutes.
3. Stir in curry powder, cooking for 1 minute until fragrant.
4. Add cauliflower and vegetable broth. Bring to a boil.
5. Reduce heat, cover, and simmer for 20 minutes, until cauliflower is tender.
6. Use an immersion blender to puree the soup until smooth.
7. Stir in coconut milk, season with salt and pepper.
8. Simmer for an additional 5 minutes.
9. Serve hot, garnished with fresh cilantro.

Nutritional Information: Calories: 240 | Protein: 5g | Carbohydrates: 20g | Fat: 18g | Fiber: 6g | Sugar: 8g

Mediterranean Quinoa Salad

Prep Time: 15 minutes | Cooking Time: 15 minutes | Servings: 4

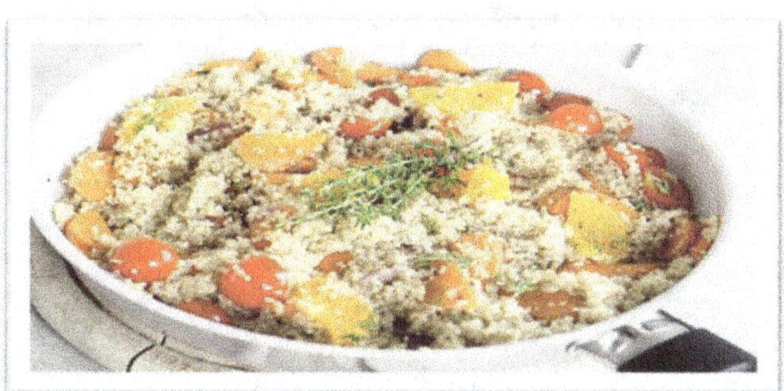

Ingredients:

- 1 cup quinoa, rinsed
- 2 cups water
- 1 cup cherry tomatoes, halved
- 1 cucumber, diced
- 1/2 red onion, finely chopped
- 1/2 cup Kalamata olives, pitted and sliced
- 1/4 cup crumbled feta cheese
- 2 tablespoons chopped fresh parsley
- 2 tablespoons olive oil
- Juice of 1 lemon
- Salt and pepper to taste

Instructions:

1. In a medium saucepan, combine quinoa and water. Bring to a boil over medium heat.
2. Reduce heat, cover, and simmer for 15 minutes, until quinoa is cooked and water is absorbed.
3. Let quinoa cool to room temperature.
4. In a large bowl, combine cooked quinoa, cherry tomatoes, cucumber, red onion, olives, feta cheese, and parsley.
5. Drizzle with olive oil and lemon juice. Season with salt and pepper.
6. Toss to combine and serve.

Nutritional Information: Calories: 250 | Protein: 8g | Carbohydrates: 32g | Fat: 10g | Fiber: 5g | Sugar: 4g

Spinach and Strawberry Salad with Walnuts

Prep Time: 10 minutes | Cooking Time: 0 minutes | Servings: 4

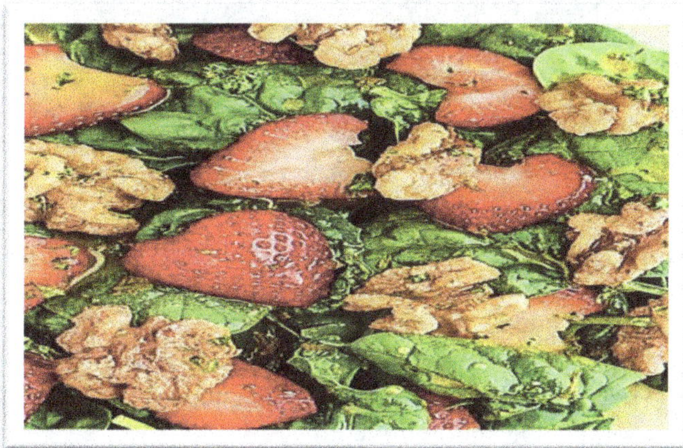

Ingredients:

- 4 cups fresh spinach
- 1 cup strawberries, sliced
- 1/4 cup walnuts, toasted and chopped
- 1/4 cup crumbled goat cheese
- 2 tablespoons balsamic vinegar
- 1 tablespoon olive oil
- 1 teaspoon honey
- Salt and pepper to taste

Instructions:

1. In a large bowl, combine spinach, strawberries, walnuts, and goat cheese.
2. In a small bowl, whisk together balsamic vinegar, olive oil, honey, salt, and pepper.
3. Drizzle dressing over salad and toss gently to combine.
4. Serve immediately.

Nutritional Information: Calories: 180 | Protein: 4g | Carbohydrates: 12g | Fat: 14g | Fiber: 3g | Sugar: 8g

Anti-Inflammatory Buddha Bowl

Prep Time: 20 minutes | Cooking Time: 30 minutes | Servings: 4

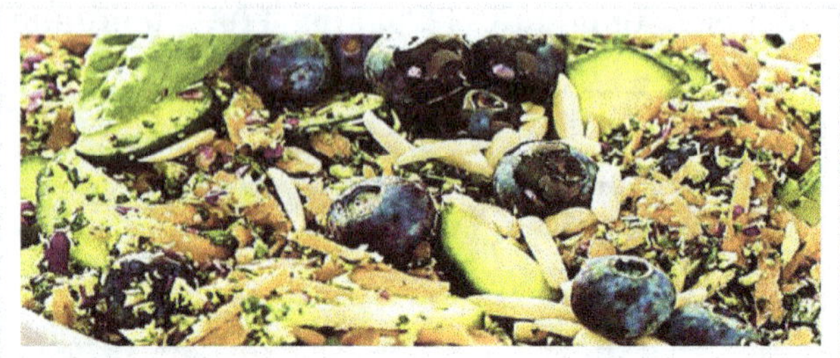

Ingredients:

- 1 cup brown rice, cooked
- 1 cup chickpeas, drained and rinsed
- 1 sweet potato, peeled and cubed
- 1 tablespoon olive oil
- 1 teaspoon ground turmeric
- 1 teaspoon ground cumin
- 2 cups spinach
- 1 avocado, sliced
- 1/4 cup tahini
- Juice of 1 lemon
- 1 garlic clove, minced
- Water, as needed for thinning
- Salt and pepper to taste

Instructions:

1. Preheat oven to 400°F (200°C).
2. Toss sweet potato cubes with olive oil, turmeric, cumin, salt, and pepper.
3. Spread on a baking sheet and roast for 25-30 minutes, until tender and golden.
4. In a large bowl, combine cooked brown rice, chickpeas, roasted sweet potato, spinach, and avocado.
5. In a small bowl, whisk together tahini, lemon juice, garlic, salt, and pepper. Add water to achieve desired consistency.
6. Drizzle dressing over the Buddha bowl and serve.

Nutritional Information: Calories: 350 | Protein: 9g | Carbohydrates: 45g | Fat: 16g | Fiber: 9g | Sugar: 4g

Chickpea and Avocado Salad

Prep Time: 10 minutes | Cooking Time: 0 minutes | Servings: 4

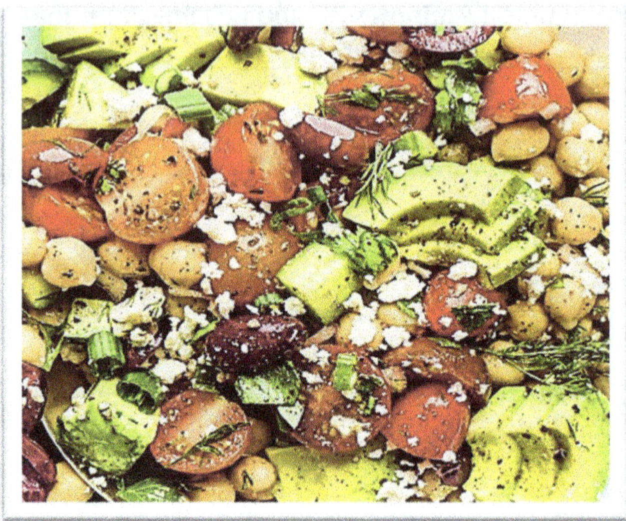

Ingredients:

- 1 can (15 oz) chickpeas, drained and rinsed
- 1 avocado, diced
- 1 cup cherry tomatoes, halved
- 1/2 red onion, finely chopped
- 1/4 cup fresh cilantro, chopped
- Juice of 1 lime
- 1 tablespoon olive oil
- Salt and pepper to taste

Instructions:

1. In a large bowl, combine chickpeas, avocado, cherry tomatoes, red onion, and cilantro.
2. Drizzle with lime juice and olive oil.
3. Season with salt and pepper.
4. Toss gently to combine and serve immediately.

Nutritional Information: Calories: 220 | Protein: 5g | Carbohydrates: 25g | Fat: 12g | Fiber: 8g | Sugar: 3g

Kale and Blueberry Superfood Salad

Prep Time: 10 minutes | Cooking Time: 0 minutes | Servings: 4

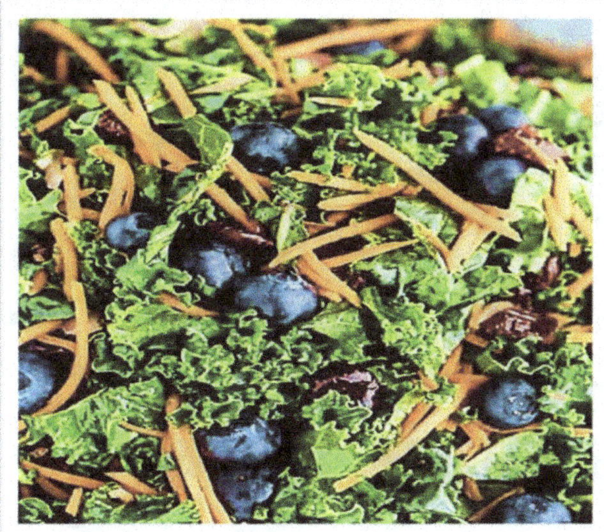

Ingredients:

- 4 cups chopped kale
- 1 cup fresh blueberries
- 1/4 cup chopped walnuts
- 1/4 cup crumbled feta cheese
- 2 tablespoons olive oil
- 1 tablespoon apple cider vinegar
- 1 teaspoon honey
- Salt and pepper to taste

Instructions:

1. In a large bowl, combine chopped kale, blueberries, walnuts, and feta cheese.
2. In a small bowl, whisk together olive oil, apple cider vinegar, honey, salt, and pepper.
3. Drizzle dressing over the salad and toss gently to combine.
4. Serve immediately.

Nutritional Information: Calories: 180 | Protein: 5g | Carbohydrates: 16g | Fat: 12g | Fiber: 4g | Sugar: 8g

Roasted Beet and Arugula Salad

Prep Time: 15 minutes | Cooking Time: 30 minutes | Servings: 4

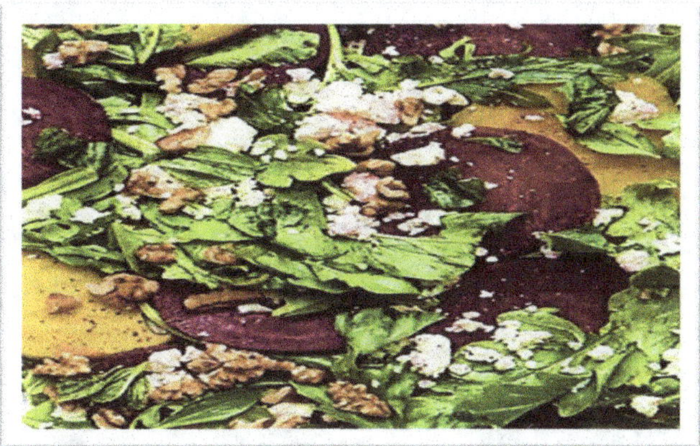

Ingredients:

- 4 medium beets, roasted and diced
- 4 cups arugula
- 1/4 cup goat cheese, crumbled
- 1/4 cup chopped pecans, toasted
- 2 tablespoons balsamic vinegar
- 1 tablespoon olive oil
- 1 teaspoon Dijon mustard
- Salt and pepper to taste

Instructions:

1. Preheat oven to 400°F (200°C). Wrap beets in aluminum foil and roast for 30 minutes, or until tender. Let cool, then peel and dice.
2. In a large bowl, combine roasted beets, arugula, goat cheese, and pecans.
3. In a small bowl, whisk together balsamic vinegar, olive oil, Dijon mustard, salt, and pepper.
4. Drizzle dressing over the salad and toss gently to combine.
5. Serve immediately.

Nutritional Information: Calories: 200 | Protein: 6g | Carbohydrates: 20g | Fat: 12g | Fiber: 5g | Sugar: 10g

Warm Lentil Salad with Lemon

Prep Time: 10 minutes | Cooking Time: 25 minutes | Servings: 4

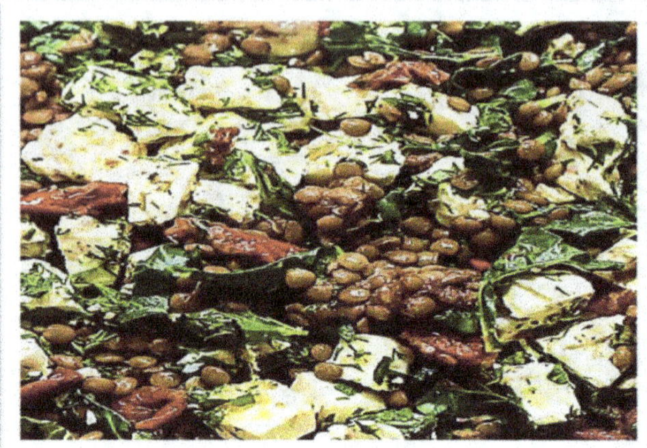

Ingredients:

- 1 cup green lentils, rinsed
- 2 cups water
- 1/2 red onion, finely chopped
- 1 cup cherry tomatoes, halved
- 1/4 cup fresh parsley, chopped
- Juice of 1 lemon
- 2 tablespoons olive oil
- Salt and pepper to taste

Instructions:

1. In a medium saucepan, combine lentils and water. Bring to a boil over medium heat.
2. Reduce heat, cover, and simmer for 20-25 minutes, until lentils are tender. Drain any excess water.
3. In a large bowl, combine cooked lentils, red onion, cherry tomatoes, and parsley.
4. Drizzle with lemon juice and olive oil.
5. Season with salt and pepper.
6. Toss gently to combine and serve warm.

Nutritional Information: Calories: 180 | Protein: 10g | Carbohydrates: 25g | Fat: 6g | Fiber: 8g | Sugar: 3g

Cucumber, Tomato, and Feta Salad

Prep Time: 10 minutes | Cooking Time: 0 minutes | Servings: 4

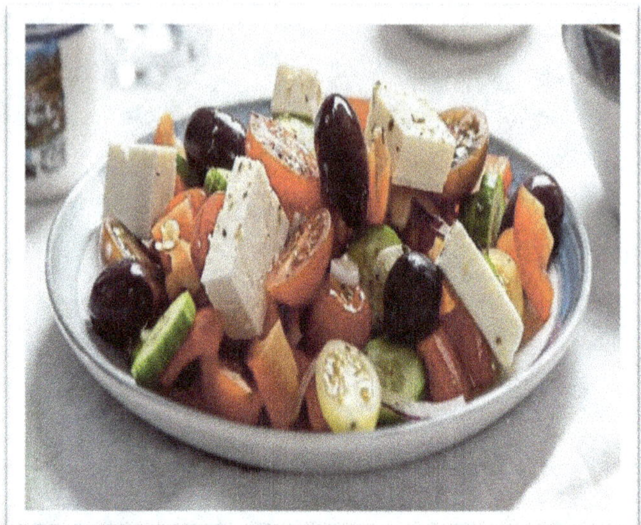

Ingredients:

- 2 cucumbers, diced
- 2 cups cherry tomatoes, halved
- 1/4 red onion, thinly sliced
- 1/4 cup crumbled feta cheese
- 2 tablespoons olive oil
- 1 tablespoon red wine vinegar
- 1 teaspoon dried oregano
- Salt and pepper to taste

Instructions:

1. In a large bowl, combine cucumbers, cherry tomatoes, red onion, and feta cheese.
2. In a small bowl, whisk together olive oil, red wine vinegar, oregano, salt, and pepper.
3. Drizzle dressing over the salad and toss gently to combine.
4. Serve immediately.

Nutritional Information: Calories: 140 | Protein: 4g | Carbohydrates: 10g | Fat: 10g | Fiber: 2g | Sugar: 5g

Baked Salmon with Lemon and Dill

Prep Time: 10 minutes | Cooking Time: 20 minutes | Servings: 4

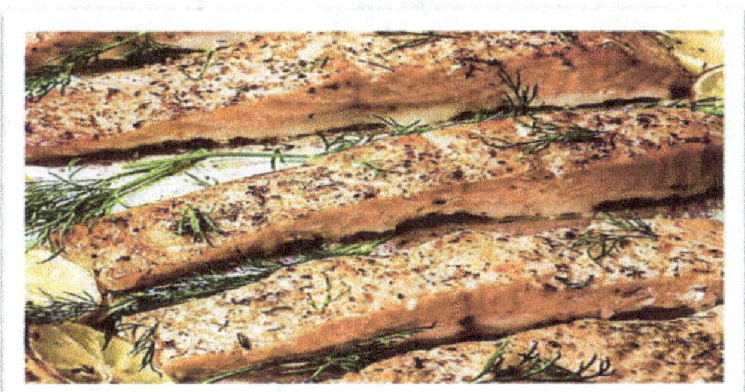

Ingredients:

- 4 salmon fillets
- 2 tablespoons olive oil
- Juice of 1 lemon
- 1 tablespoon fresh dill, chopped
- Salt and pepper to taste
- Lemon slices, for garnish

Instructions:

1. Preheat oven to 375°F (190°C).
2. Place salmon fillets on a baking sheet lined with parchment paper.
3. Drizzle olive oil and lemon juice over the salmon.
4. Sprinkle with fresh dill, salt, and pepper.
5. Bake for 15-20 minutes, until salmon is cooked through and flakes easily with a fork.
6. Garnish with lemon slices and serve.

Nutritional Information: Calories: 280 | Protein: 25g | Carbohydrates: 2g | Fat: 19g | Fiber: 0g | Sugar: 0g

Quinoa Stuffed Bell Peppers

Prep Time: 15 minutes | Cooking Time: 30 minutes | Servings: 4

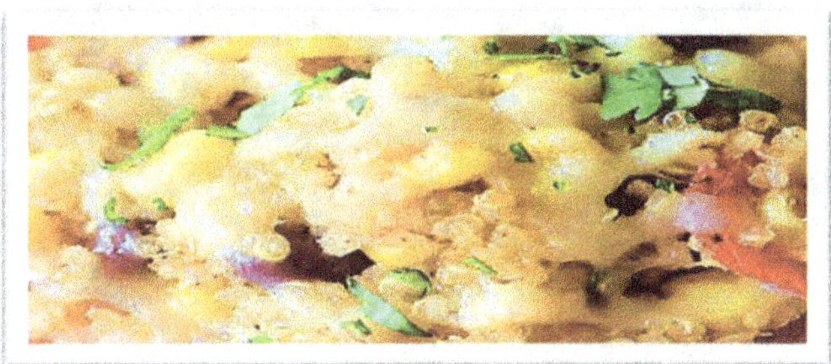

Ingredients:

- 4 bell peppers, tops cut off and seeds removed
- 1 cup quinoa, rinsed
- 2 cups vegetable broth
- 1 can (15 oz) black beans, drained and rinsed
- 1 cup corn kernels
- 1 cup diced tomatoes
- 1 teaspoon ground cumin
- 1 teaspoon chili powder
- Salt and pepper to taste
- 1/2 cup shredded cheese (optional)

Instructions:

1. Preheat oven to 375°F (190°C).
2. In a medium saucepan, bring quinoa and vegetable broth to a boil. Reduce heat, cover, and simmer for 15 minutes, until quinoa is cooked.
3. In a large bowl, combine cooked quinoa, black beans, corn, diced tomatoes, cumin, chili powder, salt, and pepper.
4. Stuff each bell pepper with the quinoa mixture and place them in a baking dish.
5. Cover with aluminum foil and bake for 25 minutes.
6. Remove foil, sprinkle with shredded cheese if using, and bake for an additional 5 minutes.
7. Serve hot.

Nutritional Information: Calories: 220 | Protein: 9g | Carbohydrates: 38g | Fat: 4g | Fiber: 10g | Sugar: 8g

Turmeric Chicken and Rice

Prep Time: 15 minutes | Cooking Time: 30 minutes | Servings: 4

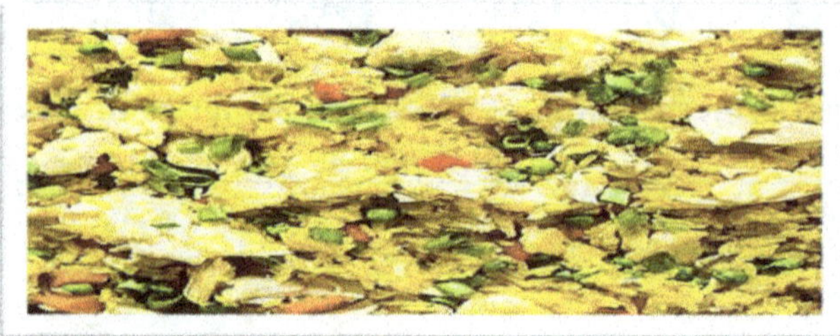

Ingredients:

- 1 tablespoon olive oil
- 1 onion, diced
- 2 cloves garlic, minced
- 1 tablespoon ground turmeric
- 1 teaspoon ground cumin
- 4 boneless, skinless chicken breasts
- 1 cup basmati rice
- 2 cups chicken broth
- 1 cup frozen peas
- Salt and pepper to taste
- Fresh cilantro, for garnish

Instructions:

1. In a large skillet, heat olive oil over medium heat.
2. Add onion and garlic, sauté until softened, about 5 minutes.
3. Stir in turmeric and cumin, cooking for 1 minute until fragrant.
4. Add chicken breasts and cook until browned on both sides, about 5 minutes per side.
5. Add rice and chicken broth to the skillet. Bring to a boil.
6. Reduce heat, cover, and simmer for 20 minutes, until chicken is cooked through and rice is tender.
7. Stir in frozen peas and cook for an additional 5 minutes.
8. Season with salt and pepper.
9. Serve hot, garnished with fresh cilantro.

Nutritional Information: Calories: 350 | Protein: 30g | Carbohydrates: 45g | Fat: 8g | Fiber: 3g | Sugar: 2g

Lentil and Vegetable Stir-Fry

Prep Time: 15 minutes | Cooking Time: 20 minutes | Servings: 4

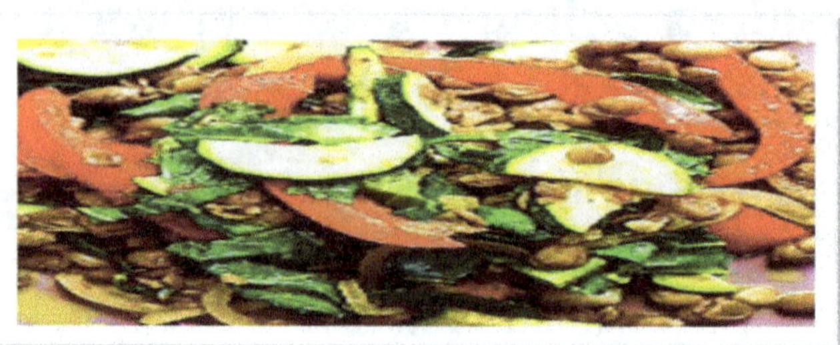

Ingredients:

- 1 tablespoon olive oil
- 1 onion, diced
- 2 cloves garlic, minced
- 1 bell pepper, sliced
- 1 zucchini, sliced
- 1 cup broccoli florets
- 1 cup cooked lentils
- 2 tablespoons soy sauce
- 1 tablespoon rice vinegar
- 1 teaspoon grated ginger
- 1/4 teaspoon red pepper flakes
- Fresh cilantro, for garnish

Instructions:

1. In a large skillet or wok, heat olive oil over medium heat.
2. Add onion and garlic, sauté until softened, about 5 minutes.
3. Add bell pepper, zucchini, and broccoli. Cook for 5-7 minutes, until vegetables are tender-crisp.
4. Stir in cooked lentils, soy sauce, rice vinegar, grated ginger, and red pepper flakes.
5. Cook for an additional 5 minutes, until heated through.
6. Serve hot, garnished with fresh cilantro.

Nutritional Information: Calories: 200 | Protein: 10g | Carbohydrates: 30g | Fat: 5g | Fiber: 10g | Sugar: 6g

Spaghetti Squash with Tomato and Basil

Prep Time: 15 minutes | Cooking Time: 45 minutes | Servings: 4

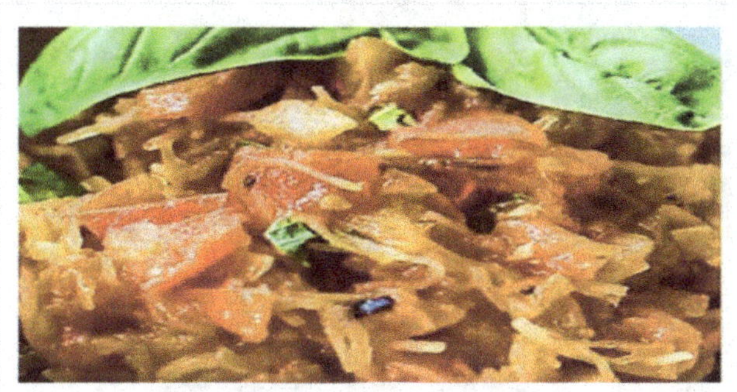

Ingredients:

- 1 large spaghetti squash
- 2 tablespoons olive oil, divided
- Salt and pepper to taste
- 1 onion, diced
- 2 cloves garlic, minced
- 1 can (14.5 oz) diced tomatoes
- 1 teaspoon dried oregano
- 1/4 cup fresh basil, chopped
- 1/4 cup grated Parmesan cheese (optional)

Instructions:

1. Preheat oven to 400°F (200°C).
2. Cut the spaghetti squash in half lengthwise and remove seeds.
3. Drizzle with 1 tablespoon olive oil, salt, and pepper.
4. Place cut side down on a baking sheet and roast for 40-45 minutes, until tender.
5. In a large skillet, heat remaining olive oil over medium heat.
6. Add onion and garlic, sauté until softened, about 5 minutes.
7. Stir in diced tomatoes and oregano, cooking for 10 minutes.
8. Use a fork to scrape the spaghetti squash strands into the skillet.
9. Toss to combine and heat through.
10. Serve hot, garnished with fresh basil and Parmesan cheese if desired.

Nutritional Information: Calories: 180 | Protein: 5g | Carbohydrates: 25g | Fat: 7g | Fiber: 5g | Sugar: 10g

Grilled Tofu with Ginger Soy Marinade

Prep Time: 10 minutes | Cooking Time: 15 minutes | Servings: 4

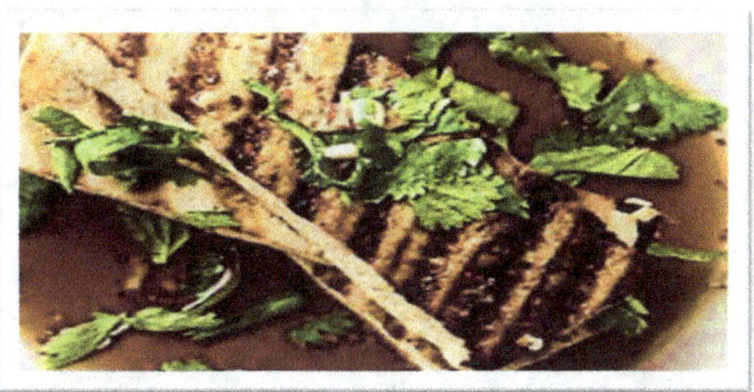

Ingredients:

- 1 block (14 oz) firm tofu, drained and pressed
- 1/4 cup soy sauce
- 2 tablespoons rice vinegar
- 1 tablespoon olive oil
- 1 tablespoon grated ginger
- 2 cloves garlic, minced
- 1 teaspoon honey
- Fresh green onions, for garnish

Instructions:

1. Cut tofu into 1/2-inch slices.
2. In a bowl, whisk together soy sauce, rice vinegar, olive oil, grated ginger, garlic, and honey.
3. Place tofu slices in a shallow dish and pour marinade over them. Let marinate for at least 30 minutes.
4. Preheat grill or grill pan over medium heat.
5. Grill tofu slices for 5-7 minutes on each side, until golden and heated through.
6. Serve hot, garnished with fresh green onions.

Nutritional Information: Calories: 150 | Protein: 10g | Carbohydrates: 8g | Fat: 10g | Fiber: 2g | Sugar: 2g

Herb-Crusted Cod

Prep Time: 10 minutes | Cooking Time: 20 minutes | Servings: 4

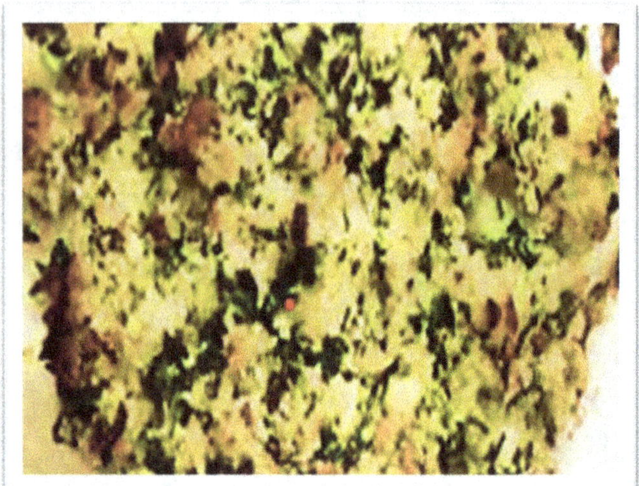

Ingredients:

- 4 cod fillets
- 2 tablespoons olive oil
- 1/4 cup fresh parsley, chopped
- 1/4 cup fresh dill, chopped
- 2 cloves garlic, minced
- Zest of 1 lemon
- Salt and pepper to taste

Instructions:

1. Preheat oven to 400°F (200°C).
2. In a small bowl, combine olive oil, parsley, dill, garlic, lemon zest, salt, and pepper.
3. Place cod fillets on a baking sheet lined with parchment paper.
4. Spread herb mixture evenly over the top of each fillet.
5. Bake for 15-20 minutes, until fish is cooked through and flakes easily with a fork.
6. Serve hot.

Nutritional Information: Calories: 200 | Protein: 25g | Carbohydrates: 2g | Fat: 10g | Fiber: 0g | Sugar: 0g

Zucchini Noodles with Pesto

Prep Time: 15 minutes | Cooking Time: 10 minutes | Servings: 4

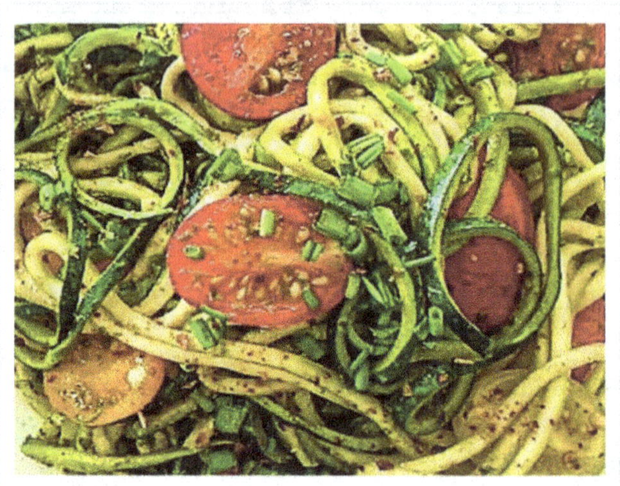

Ingredients:

- 4 zucchinis, spiralized into noodles
- 1/2 cup fresh basil leaves
- 1/4 cup pine nuts
- 2 cloves garlic
- 1/4 cup grated Parmesan cheese
- 1/4 cup olive oil
- Salt and pepper to taste

Instructions:

1. In a food processor, combine basil, pine nuts, garlic, Parmesan cheese, olive oil, salt, and pepper. Blend until smooth to make the pesto.
2. In a large skillet, heat a little olive oil over medium heat.
3. Add zucchini noodles and sauté for 3-5 minutes, until tender.
4. Remove from heat and toss with pesto.
5. Serve immediately.

Nutritional Information: Calories: 180 | Protein: 5g | Carbohydrates: 10g | Fat: 15g | Fiber: 3g | Sugar: 5g

Mushroom and Spinach Stuffed Portobellos

Prep Time: 15 minutes | Cooking Time: 20 minutes | Servings: 4

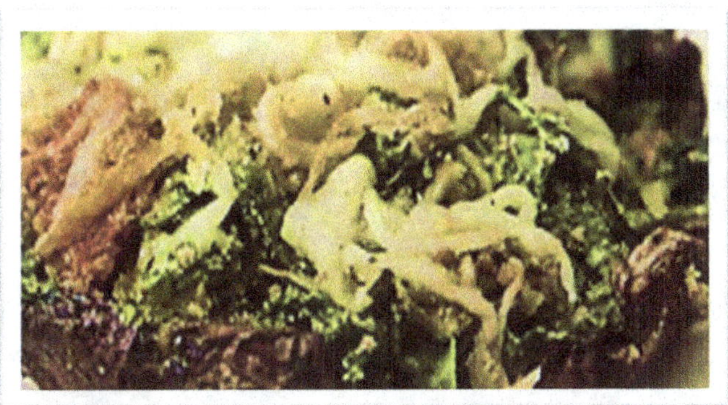

Ingredients:

- 4 large portobello mushrooms, stems removed
- 2 tablespoons olive oil, divided
- 1 onion, diced
- 2 cloves garlic, minced
- 2 cups fresh spinach
- 1 cup diced mushrooms
- 1/2 cup breadcrumbs
- 1/4 cup grated Parmesan cheese
- Salt and pepper to taste

Instructions:

1. Preheat oven to 375°F (190°C).
2. Brush portobello mushrooms with 1 tablespoon olive oil and place on a baking sheet.
3. In a large skillet, heat remaining olive oil over medium heat.
4. Add onion and garlic, sauté until softened, about 5 minutes.
5. Stir in spinach and diced mushrooms, cooking until spinach is wilted.
6. Remove from heat and stir in breadcrumbs, Parmesan cheese, salt, and pepper.
7. Stuff each portobello mushroom with the spinach mixture.
8. Bake for 20 minutes, until mushrooms are tender and stuffing is golden.
9. Serve hot.

Nutritional Information: Calories: 220 | Protein: 8g | Carbohydrates: 20g | Fat: 12g | Fiber: 4g | Sugar: 6g

Chickpea and Spinach Curry

Prep Time: 10 minutes | Cooking Time: 25 minutes | Servings: 4

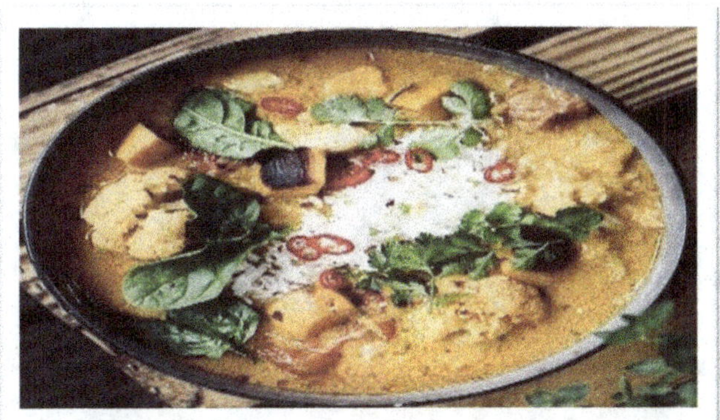

Ingredients:

- 1 tablespoon olive oil
- 1 onion, diced
- 2 cloves garlic, minced
- 1 tablespoon grated ginger
- 1 tablespoon curry powder
- 1 can (14.5 oz) diced tomatoes
- 1 can (15 oz) chickpeas, drained and rinsed
- 4 cups fresh spinach
- 1 cup coconut milk
- Salt and pepper to taste
- Fresh cilantro, for garnish

Instructions:

1. In a large skillet, heat olive oil over medium heat.
2. Add onion, garlic, and ginger, sauté until softened, about 5 minutes.
3. Stir in curry powder, cooking for 1 minute until fragrant.
4. Add diced tomatoes and chickpeas, bringing to a simmer.
5. Cook for 10 minutes, then stir in spinach and coconut milk.
6. Simmer for an additional 5 minutes, until spinach is wilted and curry is heated through.
7. Season with salt and pepper.
8. Serve hot, garnished with fresh cilantro.

Nutritional Information: Calories: 260 | Protein: 8g | Carbohydrates: 28g | Fat: 12g | Fiber: 8g | Sugar: 6g

Roasted Cauliflower Steaks

Prep Time: 10 minutes | **Cooking Time:** 30 minutes | Servings: 4

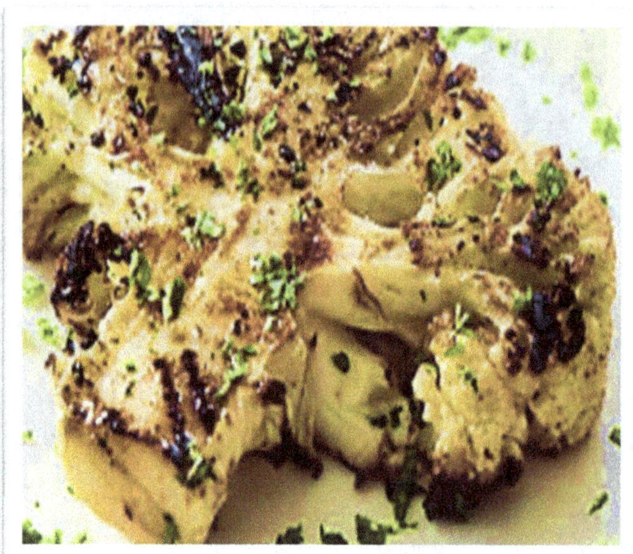

Ingredients:

- 1 large head of cauliflower
- 2 tablespoons olive oil
- 1 teaspoon ground turmeric
- 1 teaspoon ground cumin
- Salt and pepper to taste
- Fresh parsley, for garnish

Instructions:

1. Preheat oven to 400°F (200°C).
2. Cut cauliflower into thick steaks.
3. Brush both sides of each steak with olive oil.
4. Sprinkle with turmeric, cumin, salt, and pepper.
5. Place cauliflower steaks on a baking sheet and roast for 25-30 minutes, until golden and tender.
6. Serve hot, garnished with fresh parsley.

Nutritional Information: Calories: 120 | Protein: 4g | Carbohydrates: 10g | Fat: 8g | Fiber: 4g | Sugar: 3g

Baked Cod with Tomato and Olives

Prep Time: 10 minutes | **Cooking Time:** 20 minutes | Servings: 4

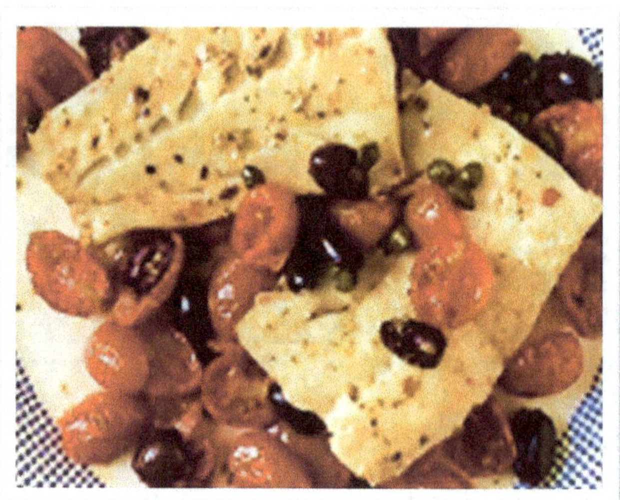

Ingredients:

- 4 cod fillets
- 2 tablespoons olive oil
- 1 cup cherry tomatoes, halved
- 1/2 cup Kalamata olives, pitted and sliced
- 2 cloves garlic, minced
- 1/4 cup fresh parsley, chopped
- Salt and pepper to taste

Instructions:

1. Preheat oven to 375°F (190°C).
2. Place cod fillets in a baking dish.
3. Drizzle with olive oil and season with salt and pepper.
4. Scatter cherry tomatoes, olives, and garlic around the fish.
5. Bake for 15-20 minutes, until cod is cooked through and flakes easily with a fork.
6. Sprinkle with fresh parsley and serve hot.

Nutritional Information: Calories: 230 | Protein: 25g | Carbohydrates: 5g | Fat: 12g | Fiber: 2g | Sugar: 3g

Sweet Potato and Black Bean Enchiladas

Prep Time: 15 minutes | Cooking Time: 30 minutes | Servings: 4

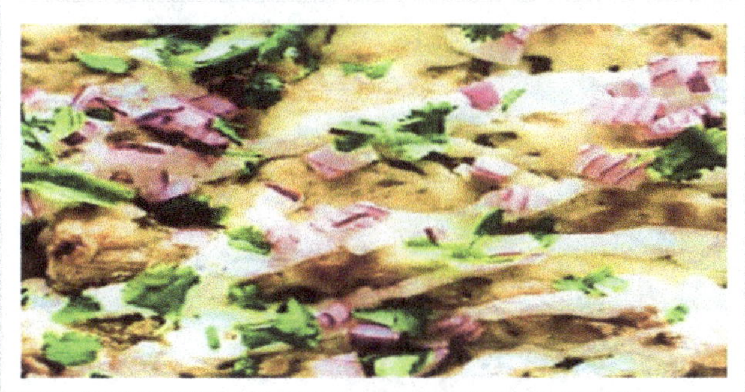

Ingredients:

- 2 large sweet potatoes, peeled and cubed
- 1 can (15 oz) black beans, drained and rinsed
- 1/2 cup corn kernels
- 1/2 cup diced tomatoes
- 1 teaspoon ground cumin
- 1 teaspoon chili powder
- Salt and pepper to taste
- 8 small whole wheat tortillas
- 1 cup enchilada sauce
- 1/2 cup shredded cheese (optional)
- Fresh cilantro, for garnish

Instructions:

1. Preheat the oven to 375°F (190°C).
2. In a large pot, boil sweet potato cubes until tender, about 10 minutes. Drain and mash.
3. In a large bowl, combine mashed sweet potatoes, black beans, corn, diced tomatoes, cumin, chili powder, salt, and pepper.
4. Spoon the mixture into each tortilla and roll up. Place seam-side down in a baking dish.
5. Pour enchilada sauce over the top and sprinkle with shredded cheese if using.
6. Bake for 20 minutes, until heated through and cheese is melted.
7. Serve hot, garnished with fresh cilantro.

Nutritional Information: Calories: 320 | Protein: 10g | Carbohydrates: 50g | Fat: 8g | Fiber: 12g | Sugar: 8g

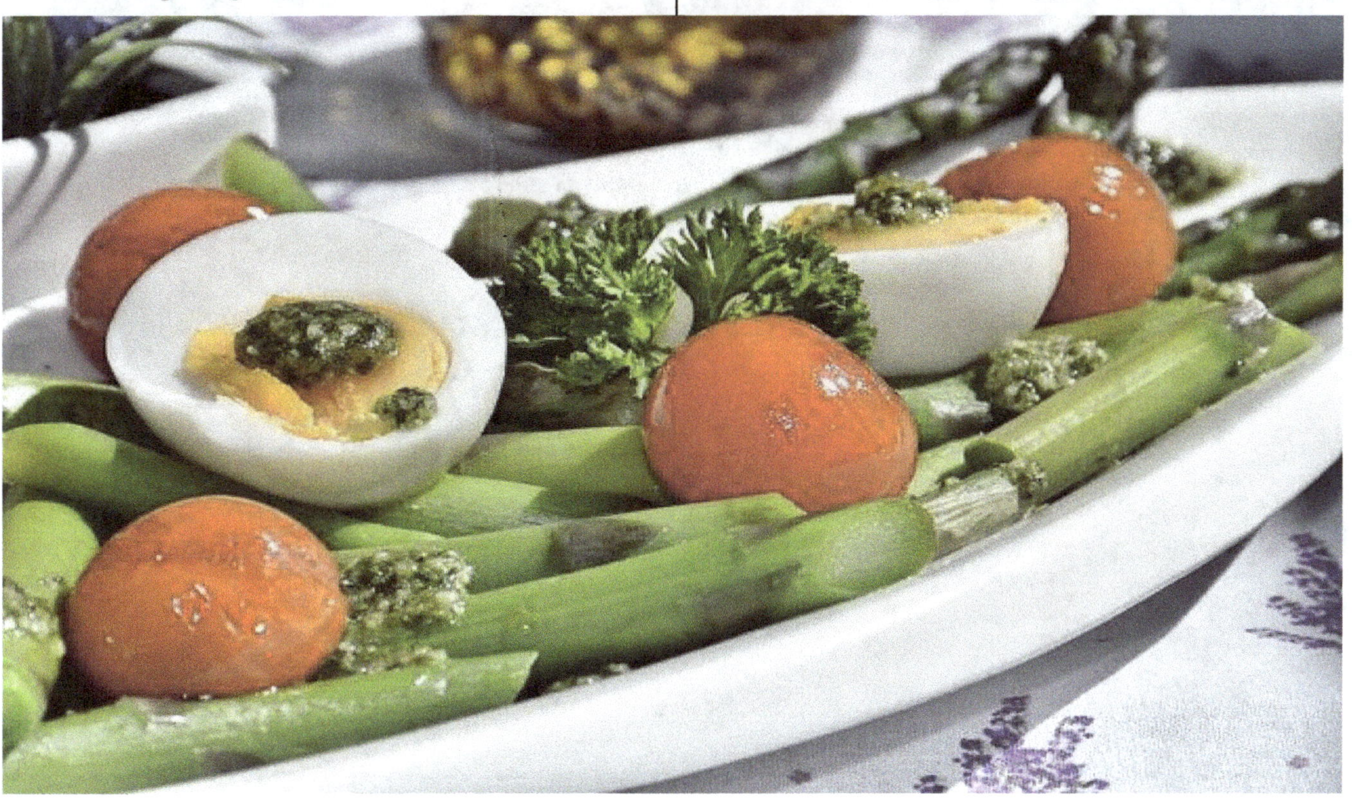

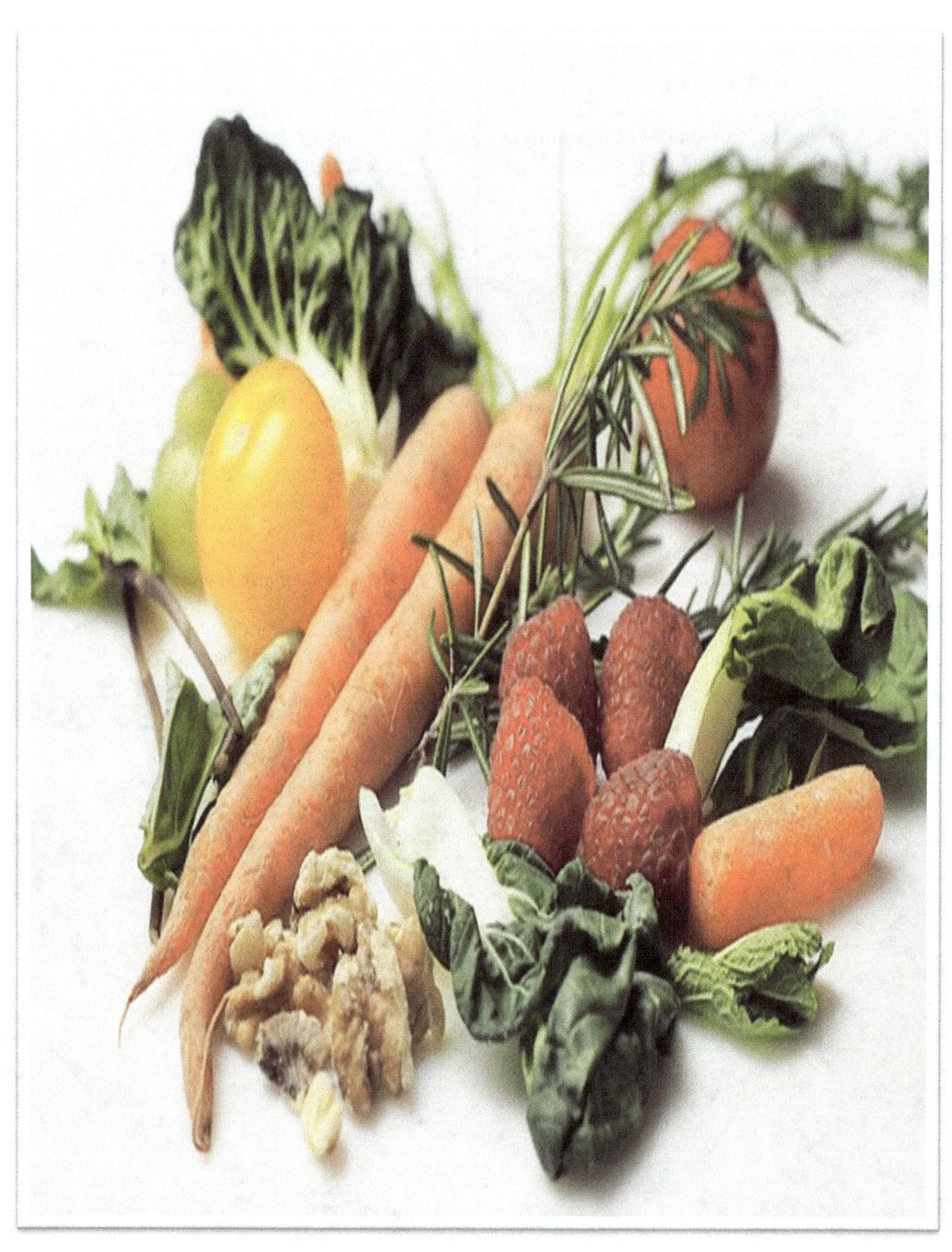

Roasted Brussels Sprouts with Balsamic Glaze

Prep Time: 10 minutes | Cooking Time: 25 minutes | Servings: 4

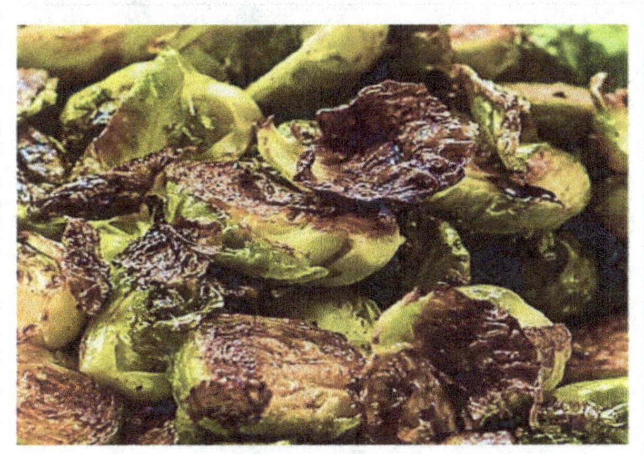

Ingredients:

- 1 pound Brussels sprouts, trimmed and halved
- 2 tablespoons olive oil
- Salt and pepper to taste
- 2 tablespoons balsamic vinegar
- 1 tablespoon honey

Instructions:

1. Preheat oven to 400°F (200°C).
2. Toss Brussels sprouts with olive oil, salt, and pepper.
3. Spread on a baking sheet and roast for 20-25 minutes, until tender and golden.
4. In a small saucepan, heat balsamic vinegar and honey over medium heat until it thickens slightly, about 2-3 minutes.
5. Drizzle balsamic glaze over roasted Brussels sprouts and serve.

Nutritional Information: Calories: 120 | Protein: 3g | Carbohydrates: 15g | Fat: 7g | Fiber: 4g | Sugar: 8g

Garlic and Herb Sweet Potato Fries

Prep Time: 10 minutes | Cooking Time: 25 minutes | Servings: 4

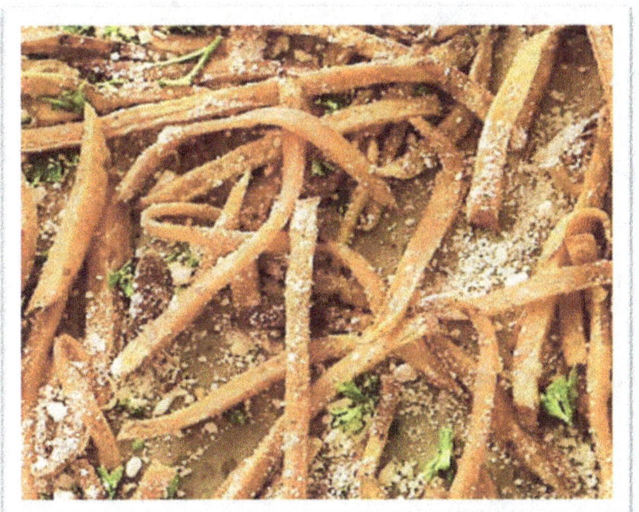

Ingredients:

- 2 large sweet potatoes, cut into fries
- 2 tablespoons olive oil
- 2 cloves garlic, minced
- 1 teaspoon dried rosemary
- 1 teaspoon dried thyme
- Salt and pepper to taste

Instructions:

1. Preheat oven to 425°F (220°C).
2. Toss sweet potato fries with olive oil, garlic, rosemary, thyme, salt, and pepper.
3. Spread on a baking sheet in a single layer.
4. Roast for 20-25 minutes, turning once, until golden and crispy.
5. Serve hot.

Nutritional Information: Calories: 150 | Protein: 2g | Carbohydrates: 26g | Fat: 6g | Fiber: 4g | Sugar: 5g

Cauliflower Rice Pilaf

Prep Time: 10 minutes | Cooking Time: 10 minutes | Servings: 4

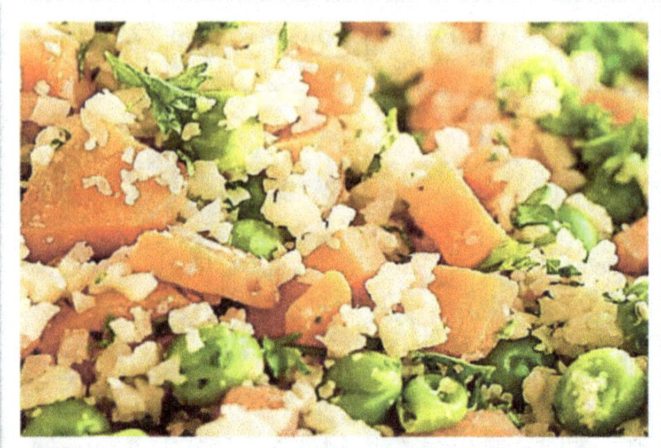

Ingredients:

- 1 large head of cauliflower, riced
- 1 tablespoon olive oil
- 1 onion, diced
- 2 cloves garlic, minced
- 1/2 cup diced carrots
- 1/2 cup peas
- 1/4 cup sliced almonds
- 1 teaspoon ground cumin
- Salt and pepper to taste

Instructions:

1. In a large skillet, heat olive oil over medium heat.
2. Add onion and garlic, sauté until softened, about 5 minutes.
3. Stir in carrots and cook for another 3 minutes.
4. Add rice cauliflower, peas, almonds, cumin, salt, and pepper.
5. Cook for an additional 5 minutes, until vegetables are tender.
6. Serve hot.

Nutritional Information: Calories: 110 | Protein: 4g | Carbohydrates: 12g | Fat: 6g | Fiber: 4g | Sugar: 4g

Steamed Asparagus with Lemon

Prep Time: 5 minutes | Cooking Time: 10 minutes | Servings: 4

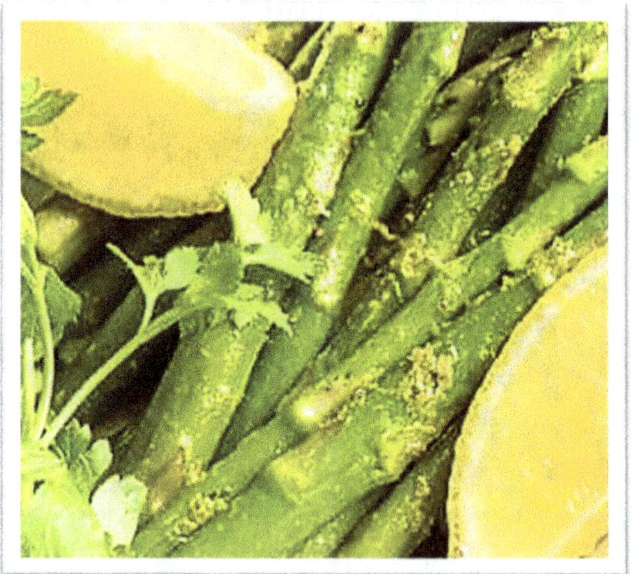

Ingredients:

- 1 bunch asparagus, trimmed
- 1 tablespoon olive oil
- Juice of 1/2 lemon
- Salt and pepper to taste
- Lemon wedges, for garnish

Instructions:

1. Steam asparagus in a steamer basket over boiling water for 5-7 minutes, until tender-crisp.
2. Remove asparagus and place on a serving platter.
3. Drizzle with olive oil and lemon juice.
4. Season with salt and pepper.
5. Serve hot, garnished with lemon wedges.

Nutritional Information: Calories: 60 | Protein: 2g | Carbohydrates: 6g | Fat: 4g | Fiber: 2g | Sugar: 2g

Turmeric Spiced Quinoa

Prep Time: 5 minutes | Cooking Time: 15 minutes | Servings: 4

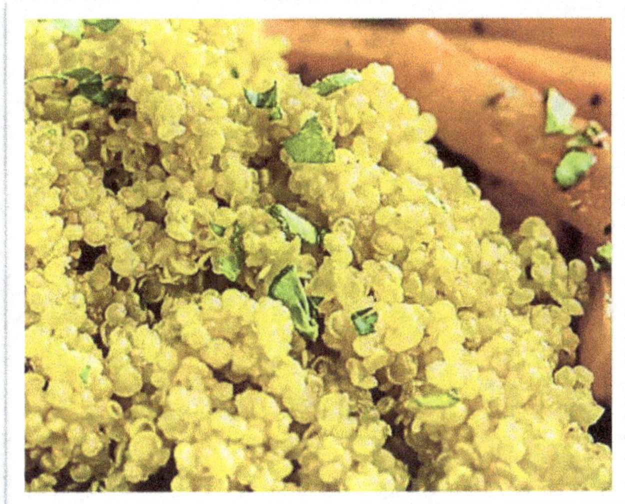

Ingredients:

- 1 cup quinoa, rinsed
- 2 cups water
- 1 tablespoon olive oil
- 1 teaspoon ground turmeric
- 1/2 teaspoon ground cumin
- Salt and pepper to taste
- Fresh cilantro, for garnish

Instructions:

1. In a medium saucepan, bring quinoa and water to a boil.
2. Reduce heat, cover, and simmer for 15 minutes, until quinoa is cooked and water is absorbed.
3. In a small bowl, mix olive oil, turmeric, cumin, salt, and pepper.
4. Fluff quinoa with a fork and stir in the spice mixture.
5. Serve hot, garnished with fresh cilantro.

Nutritional Information: Calories: 180 | Protein: 6g | Carbohydrates: 30g | Fat: 5g | Fiber: 3g | Sugar: 1g

Sautéed Green Beans with Almonds

Prep Time: 5 minutes | Cooking Time: 10 minutes | Servings: 4

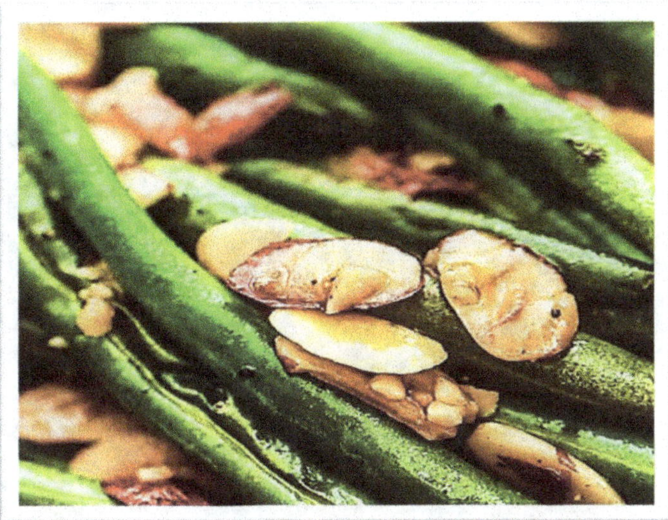

Ingredients:

- 1 pound green beans, trimmed
- 1 tablespoon olive oil
- 2 cloves garlic, minced
- 1/4 cup sliced almonds
- Salt and pepper to taste
- Lemon zest, for garnish

Instructions:

1. In a large skillet, heat olive oil over medium heat.
2. Add green beans and sauté for 5 minutes, until tender-crisp.
3. Add garlic and almonds, cooking for another 2-3 minutes until garlic is fragrant and almonds are toasted.
4. Season with salt and pepper.
5. Serve hot, garnished with lemon zest.

Nutritional Information: Calories: 120 | Protein: 3g | Carbohydrates: 10g | Fat: 8g | Fiber: 4g | Sugar: 3g

Roasted Carrot and Parsnip Medley

Prep Time: 10 minutes | Cooking Time: 30 minutes | Servings: 4

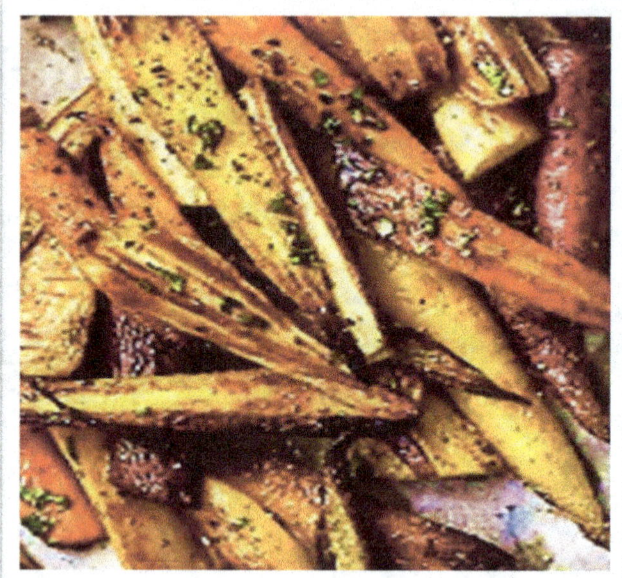

Ingredients:

- 4 large carrots, peeled and cut into sticks
- 4 parsnips, peeled and cut into sticks
- 2 tablespoons olive oil
- 1 teaspoon dried thyme
- Salt and pepper to taste
- Fresh parsley, for garnish

Instructions:

1. Preheat oven to 400°F (200°C).
2. Toss carrots and parsnips with olive oil, thyme, salt, and pepper.
3. Spread on a baking sheet in a single layer.
4. Roast for 25-30 minutes, until tender and golden.
5. Serve hot, garnished with fresh parsley.

Nutritional Information: Calories: 140 | Protein: 2g | Carbohydrates: 20g | Fat: 7g | Fiber: 6g | Sugar: 8g

Braised Red Cabbage with Apples

Prep Time: 10 minutes | Cooking Time: 30 minutes | Servings: 4

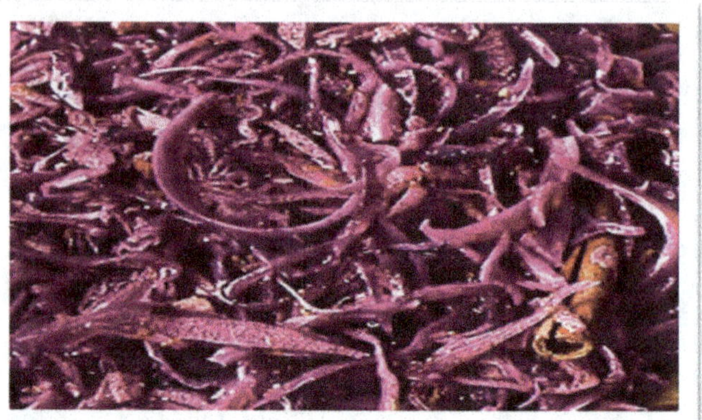

Ingredients:

- 1 tablespoon olive oil
- 1 onion, sliced
- 1 head red cabbage, thinly sliced
- 2 apples, peeled and sliced
- 1/4 cup apple cider vinegar
- 2 tablespoons honey
- Salt and pepper to taste

Instructions:

1. In a large pot, heat olive oil over medium heat.
2. Add onion and sauté until softened, about 5 minutes.
3. Stir in red cabbage and apples, cooking for another 5 minutes.
4. Add apple cider vinegar and honey, stirring to combine.
5. Cover and simmer for 20 minutes, until cabbage and apples are tender.
6. Season with salt and pepper.
7. Serve hot.

Nutritional Information: Calories: 120 | Protein: 2g | Carbohydrates: 25g | Fat: 3g | Fiber: 5g | Sugar: 18g

Vegan Lentil Loaf

Prep Time: 15 minutes | Cooking Time: 60 minutes | Servings: 4

Ingredients:

- 1 cup dry lentils, rinsed
- 2 1/2 cups water
- 1 tablespoon olive oil
- 1 onion, diced
- 2 cloves garlic, minced
- 1 carrot, grated
- 1 celery stalk, finely chopped
- 1 cup rolled oats
- 1/2 cup breadcrumbs
- 2 tablespoons ground flaxseed mixed with 6 tablespoons water
- 1/4 cup ketchup
- 2 tablespoons soy sauce
- 1 teaspoon dried thyme
- Salt and pepper to taste

Instructions:

1. Preheat oven to 350°F (175°C). Grease a loaf pan.
2. In a medium pot, bring lentils and water to a boil. Reduce heat, cover, and simmer for 30 minutes, until lentils are soft. Drain any excess water.
3. In a skillet, heat olive oil over medium heat. Add onion, garlic, carrot, and celery, sauté until vegetables are softened, about 5-7 minutes.
4. In a large bowl, combine cooked lentils, sautéed vegetables, oats, breadcrumbs, flaxseed mixture, ketchup, soy sauce, thyme, salt, and pepper. Mix well.
5. Press the mixture into the prepared loaf pan and smooth the top.
6. Bake for 45-50 minutes, until firm and golden brown.
7. Let cool slightly before slicing and serving.

Nutritional Information: Calories: 280 | Protein: 12g | Carbohydrates: 45g | Fat: 6g | Fiber: 12g | Sugar: 8g

Chickpea and Sweet Potato Buddha Bowl

Prep Time: 20 minutes | Cooking Time: 25 minutes | Servings: 4

Ingredients:

- 2 large sweet potatoes, peeled and cubed
- 1 tablespoon olive oil
- 1 teaspoon ground cumin
- 1 teaspoon smoked paprika
- Salt and pepper to taste
- 1 can (15 oz) chickpeas, drained and rinsed
- 4 cups mixed greens
- 1 avocado, sliced
- 1/4 cup tahini
- Juice of 1 lemon
- 1 clove garlic, minced
- Water, as needed for thinning

Instructions:

1. Preheat oven to 400°F (200°C).
2. Toss sweet potato cubes with olive oil, cumin, smoked paprika, salt, and pepper. Spread on a baking sheet and roast for 25 minutes, until tender.
3. In a large bowl, combine mixed greens, roasted sweet potatoes, chickpeas, and avocado slices.
4. In a small bowl, whisk together tahini, lemon juice, garlic, salt, and pepper. Add water to achieve desired consistency.
5. Drizzle dressing over the Buddha bowl and serve.

Nutritional Information: Calories: 350 | Protein: 9g | Carbohydrates: 45g | Fat: 16g | Fiber: 11g | Sugar: 7g

Cauliflower Tacos with Avocado Lime Sauce

Prep Time: 15 minutes | **Cooking Time:** 20 minutes | Servings: 4

Ingredients:

- 1 head cauliflower, cut into small florets
- 2 tablespoons olive oil
- 1 teaspoon ground cumin
- 1 teaspoon smoked paprika
- 1/2 teaspoon chili powder
- Salt and pepper to taste
- 8 small corn tortillas
- 1/4 cup chopped fresh cilantro

Avocado Lime Sauce:

- 1 ripe avocado
- Juice of 1 lime
- 1/4 cup fresh cilantro
- 1 clove garlic
- 1/4 cup water
- Salt to taste

Instructions:

1. Preheat oven to 400°F (200°C).
2. Toss cauliflower florets with olive oil, cumin, smoked paprika, chili powder, salt, and pepper. Spread on a baking sheet and roast for 20 minutes, until tender and golden.
3. In a blender, combine avocado, lime juice, cilantro, garlic, water, and salt. Blend until smooth.
4. Warm corn tortillas in a dry skillet over medium heat.
5. Fill each tortilla with roasted cauliflower and top with avocado lime sauce and chopped fresh cilantro.
6. Serve immediately.

Nutritional Information: Calories: 280 | Protein: 6g | Carbohydrates: 32g | Fat: 16g | Fiber: 10g | Sugar: 4g

Eggplant and Chickpea Stew

Prep Time: 10 minutes | **Cooking Time:** 30 minutes | Servings: 4

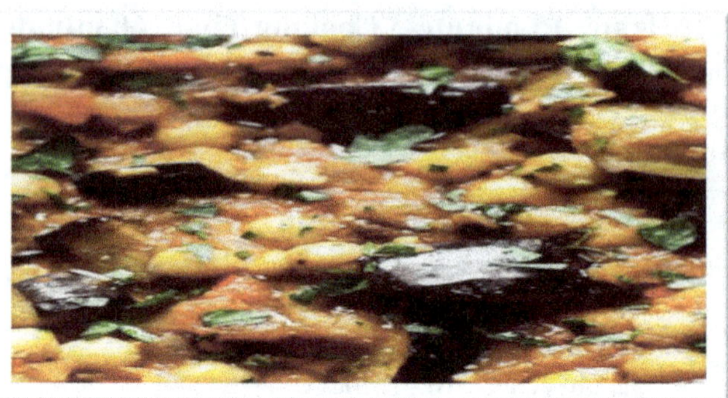

Ingredients:

- 2 tablespoons olive oil
- 1 onion, diced
- 2 cloves garlic, minced
- 1 eggplant, diced
- 1 can (15 oz) chickpeas, drained and rinsed
- 1 can (14.5 oz) diced tomatoes
- 1 teaspoon ground cumin
- 1 teaspoon smoked paprika
- 1/2 teaspoon ground cinnamon
- Salt and pepper to taste
- Fresh parsley, for garnish

Instructions:

1. In a large pot, heat olive oil over medium heat. Add onion and garlic, sauté until softened, about 5 minutes.
2. Add diced eggplant and cook for another 5 minutes, until eggplant begins to soften.
3. Stir in chickpeas, diced tomatoes, cumin, smoked paprika, cinnamon, salt, and pepper.
4. Bring to a simmer, cover, and cook for 20 minutes, until eggplant is tender.
5. Serve hot, garnished with fresh parsley.

Nutritional Information: Calories: 220 | Protein: 6g | Carbohydrates: 30g | Fat: 10g | Fiber: 8g | Sugar: 10g

Vegan Stuffed Peppers

Prep Time: 15 minutes | Cooking Time: 30 minutes | Servings: 4

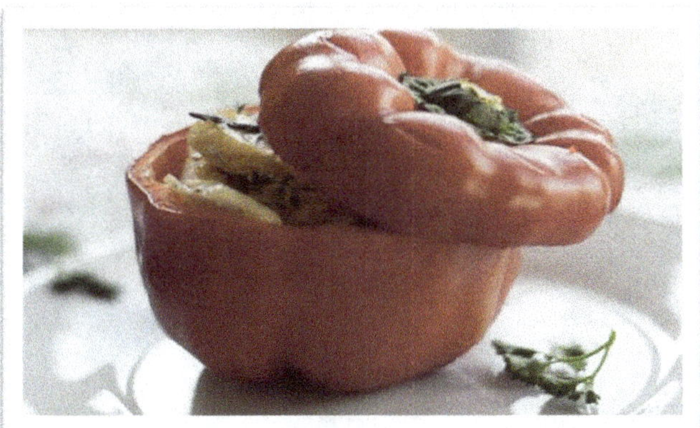

Ingredients:

- 4 bell peppers, tops cut off and seeds removed
- 1 cup quinoa, rinsed
- 2 cups vegetable broth
- 1 can (15 oz) black beans, drained and rinsed
- 1 cup corn kernels
- 1 cup diced tomatoes
- 1 teaspoon ground cumin
- 1 teaspoon chili powder
- Salt and pepper to taste
- 1/2 cup salsa (optional)

Instructions:

1. Preheat oven to 375°F (190°C).
2. In a medium saucepan, bring quinoa and vegetable broth to a boil. Reduce heat, cover, and simmer for 15 minutes, until quinoa is cooked.
3. In a large bowl, combine cooked quinoa, black beans, corn, diced tomatoes, cumin, chili powder, salt, and pepper.
4. Stuff each bell pepper with the quinoa mixture and place them in a baking dish.
5. Pour salsa over the stuffed peppers if using.
6. Cover with aluminum foil and bake for 25-30 minutes, until peppers are tender.
7. Serve hot.

Nutritional Information: Calories: 250 | Protein: 10g | Carbohydrates: 45g | Fat: 4g | Fiber: 10g | Sugar: 8g

Black Bean and Quinoa Salad

Prep Time: 15 minutes | Cooking Time: 15 minutes | Servings: 4

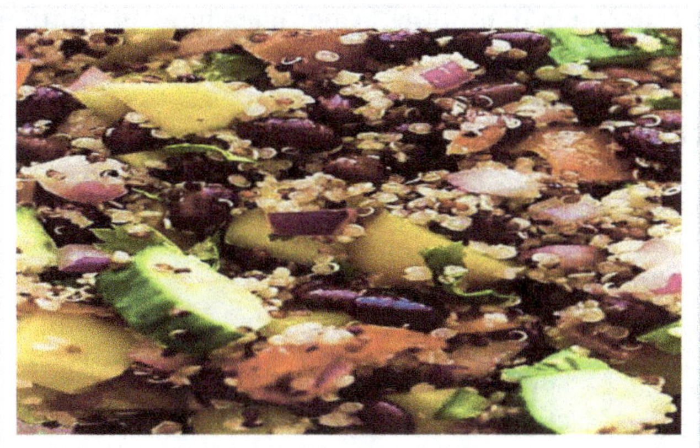

Ingredients:

- 1 cup quinoa, rinsed
- 2 cups water
- 1 can (15 oz) black beans, drained and rinsed
- 1 cup corn kernels
- 1 red bell pepper, diced
- 1/4 cup fresh cilantro, chopped
- 1/4 cup lime juice
- 2 tablespoons olive oil
- Salt and pepper to taste

Instructions:

1. In a medium saucepan, bring quinoa and water to a boil. Reduce heat, cover, and simmer for 15 minutes, until quinoa is cooked.
2. In a large bowl, combine cooked quinoa, black beans, corn, red bell pepper, and cilantro.
3. In a small bowl, whisk together lime juice, olive oil, salt, and pepper.
4. Pour dressing over the salad and toss to combine.
5. Serve immediately or refrigerate until ready to serve.

Nutritional Information: Calories: 220 | Protein: 8g | Carbohydrates: 35g | Fat: 6g | Fiber: 8g | Sugar: 4g

Sweet Potato and Lentil Shepherd's Pie

Prep Time: 20 minutes | Cooking Time: 40 minutes | Servings: 4

Ingredients:

- 2 large sweet potatoes, peeled and cubed
- 1 tablespoon olive oil
- 1 onion, diced
- 2 cloves garlic, minced
- 2 carrots, diced
- 1 cup green lentils, rinsed
- 2 cups vegetable broth
- 1 teaspoon dried thyme
- 1 teaspoon dried rosemary
- Salt and pepper to taste
- 1/4 cup almond milk

Instructions:

1. Preheat oven to 375°F (190°C).
2. In a large pot, boil sweet potato cubes until tender, about 10 minutes. Drain and mash with almond milk. Set aside.
3. In a large skillet, heat olive oil over medium heat. Add onion, garlic, and carrots, sauté until softened, about 5-7 minutes.
4. Stir in lentils, vegetable broth, thyme, rosemary, salt, and pepper. Bring to a boil, reduce heat, and simmer for 20 minutes, until lentils are tender and broth is absorbed.
5. Transfer lentil mixture to a baking dish and spread mashed sweet potatoes on top.
6. Bake for 20 minutes, until the top is slightly golden.
7. Serve hot.

Nutritional Information: Calories: 300 | Protein: 12g | Carbohydrates: 50g | Fat: 6g | Fiber: 15g | Sugar: 10g

Vegan Mushroom Stroganoff

Prep Time: 15 minutes | Cooking Time: 20 minutes | Servings: 4

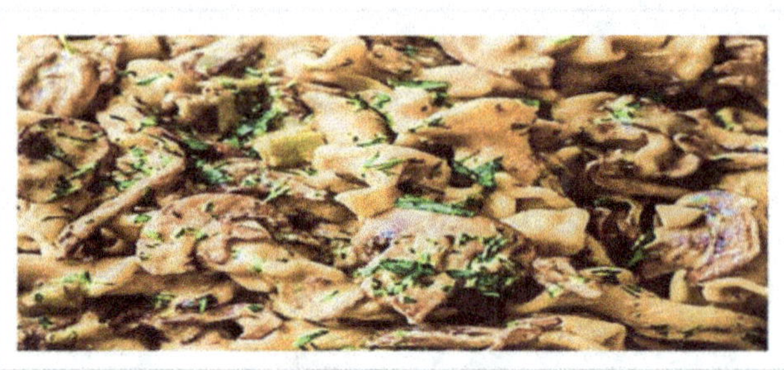

Ingredients:

- 2 tablespoons olive oil
- 1 onion, diced
- 3 cloves garlic, minced
- 1 pound mushrooms, sliced
- 1 teaspoon smoked paprika
- 1 teaspoon dried thyme
- 1/4 cup white wine (optional)
- 1 cup vegetable broth
- 1 cup coconut milk
- 2 tablespoons cornstarch mixed with 2 tablespoons water
- Salt and pepper to taste
- Fresh parsley, for garnish

Instructions:

1. In a large skillet, heat olive oil over medium heat. Add onion and garlic, sauté until softened, about 5 minutes.
2. Add mushrooms, smoked paprika, and thyme. Cook for another 5-7 minutes, until mushrooms are browned.
3. Pour in white wine (if using) and cook until evaporated.
4. Stir in vegetable broth and coconut milk. Bring to a simmer.
5. Add cornstarch mixture and cook until the sauce thickens, about 3 minutes.
6. Season with salt and pepper.
7. Serve hot, garnished with fresh parsley.

Nutritional Information: Calories: 280 | Protein: 6g | Carbohydrates: 20g | Fat: 20g | Fiber: 4g | Sugar: 6g

Blueberry Chia Pudding

Prep Time: 10 minutes | Cooking Time: 0 minutes (plus overnight chilling) | Servings: 4

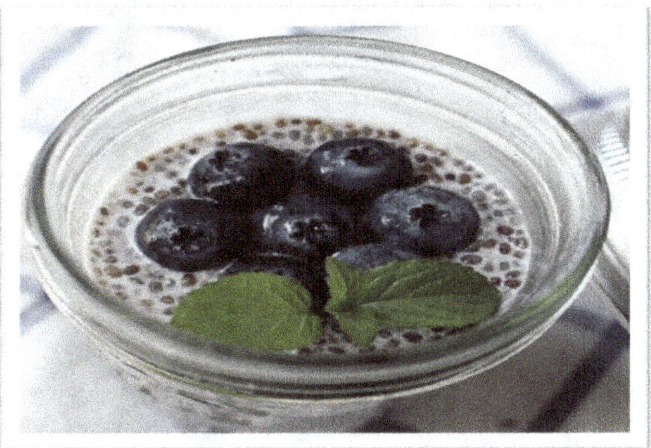

Ingredients:

- 1/4 cup chia seeds
- 1 cup unsweetened almond milk
- 1 tablespoon honey
- 1/2 teaspoon vanilla extract
- 1 cup fresh blueberries

Instructions:

1. In a medium bowl, combine chia seeds, almond milk, honey, and vanilla extract. Stir well to combine.
2. Cover and refrigerate overnight or for at least 4 hours.
3. Stir the pudding to break up any clumps before serving.
4. Divide into four bowls and top with fresh blueberries.

Nutritional Information: Calories: 120 | Protein: 3g | Carbohydrates: 19g | Fat: 5g | Fiber: 6g | Sugar: 10g

Coconut and Mango Sorbet

Prep Time: 15 minutes | Cooking Time: 0 minutes (plus freezing time) | Servings: 4

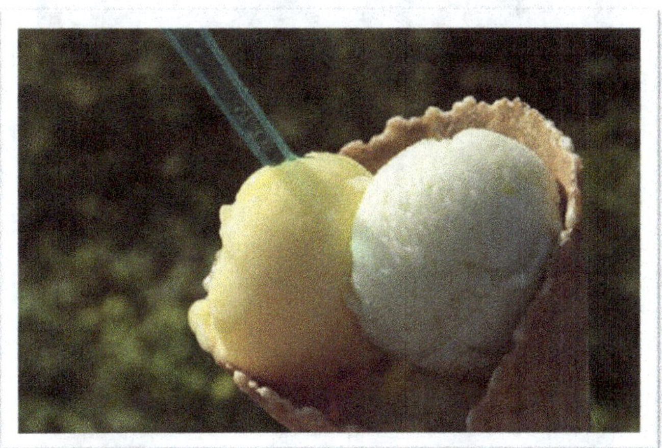

Ingredients:

- 2 ripe mangoes, peeled and diced
- 1 cup coconut milk
- 1/4 cup honey
- Juice of 1 lime

Instructions:

1. In a blender, combine mangoes, coconut milk, honey, and lime juice. Blend until smooth.
2. Pour the mixture into an ice cream maker and churn according to the manufacturer's instructions.
3. Transfer to a container and freeze for at least 2 hours before serving.

Nutritional Information: Calories: 180 | Protein: 2g | Carbohydrates: 38g | Fat: 6g | Fiber: 2g | Sugar: 32g

Dark Chocolate Avocado Mousse

Prep Time: 10 minutes | Cooking Time: 0 minutes | Servings: 4

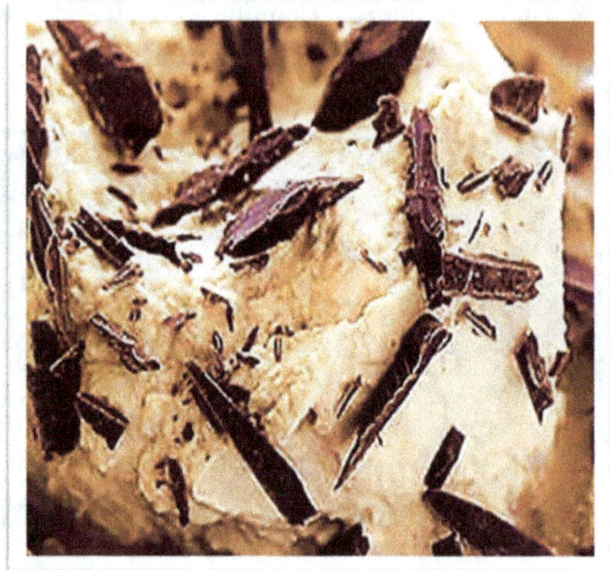

Ingredients:

- 2 ripe avocados
- 1/4 cup unsweetened cocoa powder
- 1/4 cup honey
- 1/4 cup almond milk
- 1 teaspoon vanilla extract
- Pinch of salt

Instructions:

1. In a blender or food processor, combine avocados, cocoa powder, honey, almond milk, vanilla extract, and salt. Blend until smooth and creamy.
2. Divide the mousse into four serving dishes.
3. Refrigerate for at least 30 minutes before serving.

Nutritional Information: Calories: 220 | Protein: 3g | Carbohydrates: 25g | Fat: 15g | Fiber: 8g | Sugar: 16g

Baked Apples with Cinnamon and Walnuts

Prep Time: 10 minutes | Cooking Time: 30 minutes | Servings: 4

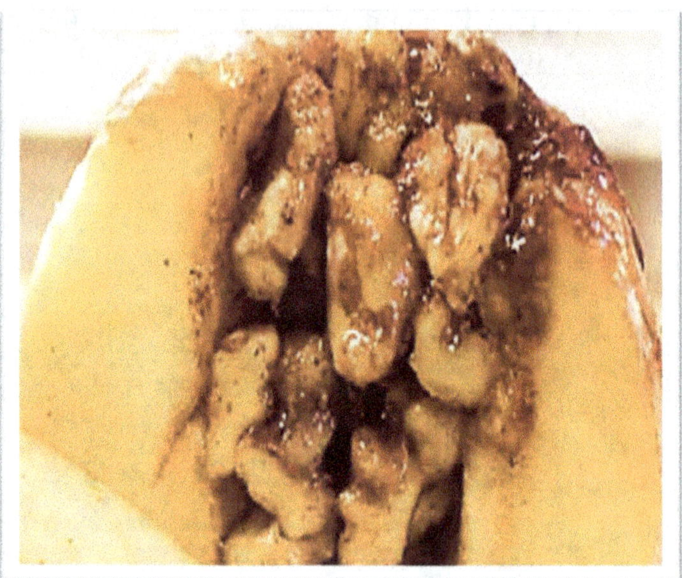

Ingredients:

- 4 large apples, cored
- 1/4 cup chopped walnuts
- 2 tablespoons honey
- 1 teaspoon ground cinnamon
- 1/2 teaspoon ground nutmeg

Instructions:

1. Preheat oven to 350°F (175°C).
2. Place cored apples in a baking dish.
3. In a small bowl, combine walnuts, honey, cinnamon, and nutmeg. Stuff the mixture into the center of each apple.
4. Bake for 25-30 minutes, until apples are tender.
5. Serve warm.

Nutritional Information: Calories: 150 | Protein: 2g | Carbohydrates: 32g | Fat: 5g | Fiber: 6g | Sugar: 24g

Turmeric and Ginger Spiced Cookies

Prep Time: 15 minutes | Cooking Time: 12 minutes | Servings: 24 cookies

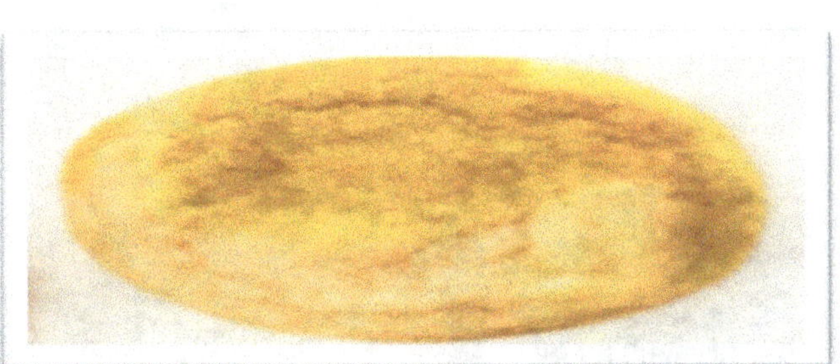

Ingredients:

- 1 1/2 cups almond flour
- 1/2 cup coconut flour
- 1/2 teaspoon baking soda
- 1 teaspoon ground turmeric
- 1 teaspoon ground ginger
- 1/4 teaspoon ground cinnamon
- 1/4 teaspoon salt
- 1/4 cup coconut oil, melted
- 1/4 cup honey
- 2 eggs
- 1 teaspoon vanilla extract

Instructions:

1. Preheat oven to 350°F (175°C). Line a baking sheet with parchment paper.
2. In a large bowl, combine almond flour, coconut flour, baking soda, turmeric, ginger, cinnamon, and salt.
3. In another bowl, whisk together melted coconut oil, honey, eggs, and vanilla extract.
4. Add wet ingredients to dry ingredients and mix until well combined.
5. Scoop tablespoon-sized balls of dough onto the prepared baking sheet, flattening them slightly.
6. Bake for 10-12 minutes, until golden brown.
7. Let cool on a wire rack before serving.

Nutritional Information: Calories: 90 | Protein: 2g | Carbohydrates: 7g | Fat: 7g | Fiber: 2g | Sugar: 4g

Berry and Almond Parfait

Prep Time: 10 minutes | Cooking Time: 0 minutes | Servings: 4

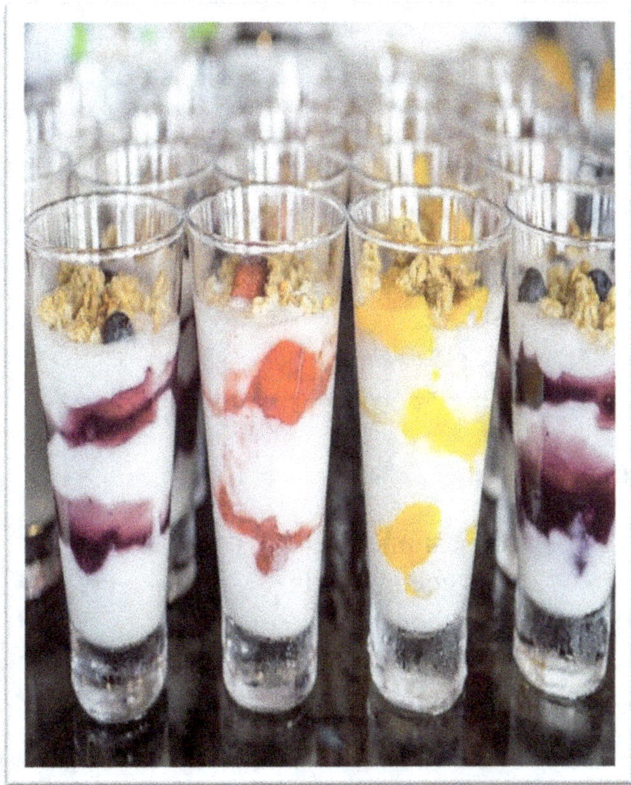

Ingredients:

- 2 cups Greek yogurt
- 1 cup mixed berries (strawberries, blueberries, raspberries)
- 1/4 cup sliced almonds
- 2 tablespoons honey

Instructions:

1. In four serving glasses, layer Greek yogurt, mixed berries, and sliced almonds.
2. Drizzle each parfait with honey.
3. Serve immediately.

Nutritional Information: Calories: 180 | Protein: 8g | Carbohydrates: 20g | Fat: 7g | Fiber: 3g | Sugar: 15g

Chilled Coconut Rice Pudding

Prep Time: 10 minutes | **Cooking Time:** 25 minutes | **Servings:** 4

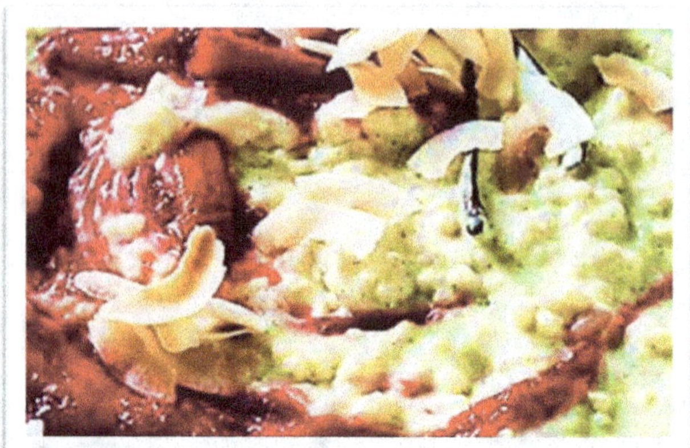

Ingredients:

- 1 cup jasmine rice
- 2 cups coconut milk
- 1/4 cup honey
- 1 teaspoon vanilla extract
- 1/4 teaspoon salt
- Fresh mango slices, for garnish

Instructions:

1. In a medium saucepan, combine jasmine rice, coconut milk, honey, vanilla extract, and salt.
2. Bring to a boil over medium heat, then reduce heat and simmer for 20-25 minutes, stirring occasionally, until rice is tender and mixture is creamy.
3. Remove from heat and let cool.
4. Refrigerate for at least 1 hour before serving.
5. Serve chilled, topped with fresh mango slices.

Nutritional Information: Calories: 250 | Protein: 4g | Carbohydrates: 45g | Fat: 6g | Fiber: 1g | Sugar: 18g

Matcha Green Tea Ice Cream

Prep Time: 15 minutes | **Cooking Time:** 0 minutes (plus freezing time) | **Servings:** 4

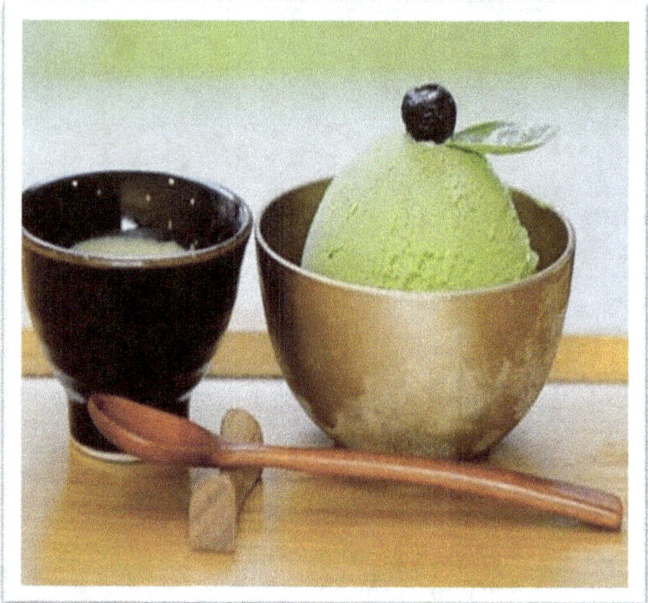

Ingredients:

- 2 cups coconut milk
- 1/2 cup honey
- 1 tablespoon matcha green tea powder
- 1 teaspoon vanilla extract

Instructions:

1. In a blender, combine coconut milk, honey, matcha green tea powder, and vanilla extract. Blend until smooth.
2. Pour the mixture into an ice cream maker and churn according to the manufacturer's instructions.
3. Transfer to a container and freeze for at least 2 hours before serving.

Nutritional Information: Calories: 220 | Protein: 2g | Carbohydrates: 30g | Fat: 11g | Fiber: 1g | Sugar: 25g

Anti-Inflammatory Golden Milk

Prep Time: 5 minutes | Cooking Time: 5 minutes | Servings: 2

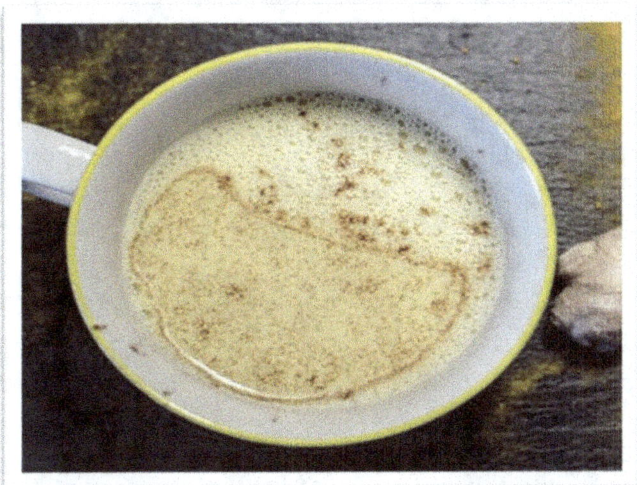

Ingredients:

- 2 cups unsweetened almond milk
- 1 teaspoon ground turmeric
- 1/2 teaspoon ground cinnamon
- 1/2 teaspoon ground ginger
- 1 tablespoon honey
- 1/2 teaspoon vanilla extract
- Pinch of black pepper

Instructions:

1. In a small saucepan, combine almond milk, turmeric, cinnamon, ginger, honey, vanilla extract, and black pepper.
2. Heat over medium heat, stirring continuously until warm (do not boil).
3. Pour into mugs and serve immediately.

Nutritional Information: Calories: 90 | Protein: 1g | Carbohydrates: 16g | Fat: 2g | Fiber: 1g | Sugar: 12g

Green Tea with Lemon and Ginger

Prep Time: 5 minutes | Cooking Time: 5 minutes | Servings: 2

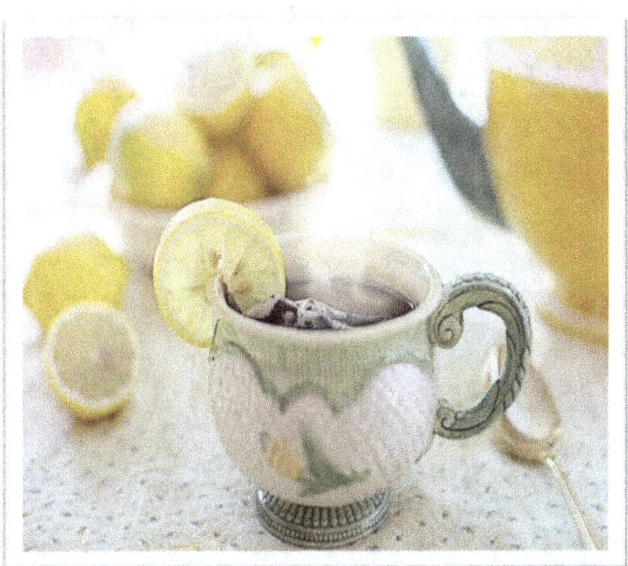

Ingredients:

- 2 cups water
- 2 green tea bags
- 1-inch piece of fresh ginger, sliced
- Juice of 1/2 lemon
- Honey to taste

Instructions:

1. In a small saucepan, bring water to a boil.
2. Remove from heat and add green tea bags and ginger slices. Steep for 3-5 minutes.
3. Remove tea bags and ginger slices.
4. Stir in lemon juice and honey to taste.
5. Pour into mugs and serve hot.

Nutritional Information: Calories: 20 | Protein: 0g | Carbohydrates: 5g | Fat: 0g | Fiber: 0g | Sugar: 5g

Berry and Mint Infused Water

Prep Time: 5 minutes | Cooking Time: 0 minutes | Servings: 4

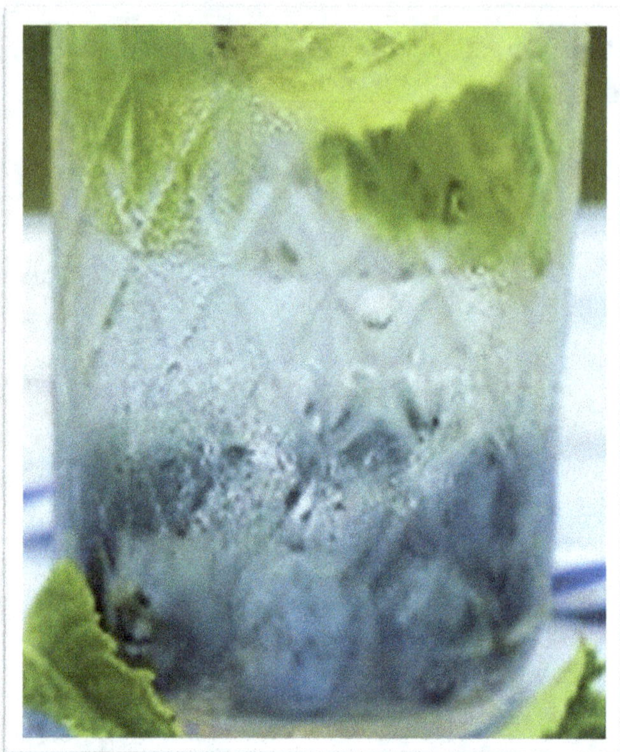

Ingredients:

- 1 cup mixed berries (strawberries, blueberries, raspberries)
- 1/4 cup fresh mint leaves
- 1 quart water
- Ice cubes

Instructions:

1. In a large pitcher, combine mixed berries and fresh mint leaves.
2. Pour water over the berries and mint.
3. Add ice cubes and stir to combine.
4. Refrigerate for at least 1 hour before serving to allow flavors to infuse.

Nutritional Information: Calories: 5 | Protein: 0g | Carbohydrates: 1g | Fat: 0g | Fiber: 0g | Sugar: 1g

Turmeric and Honey Tea

Prep Time: 5 minutes | Cooking Time: 5 minutes | Servings: 2

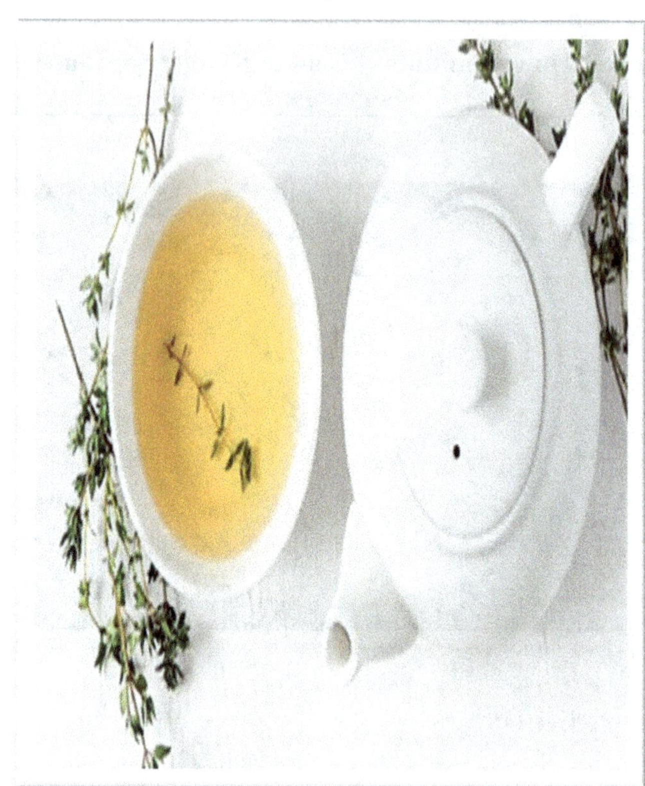

Ingredients:

- 2 cups water
- 1 teaspoon ground turmeric
- 1 tablespoon honey
- Juice of 1/2 lemon
- Pinch of black pepper

Instructions:

1. In a small saucepan, bring water to a boil.
2. Remove from heat and stir in turmeric, honey, lemon juice, and black pepper.
3. Pour into mugs and serve hot.

Nutritional Information: Calories: 30 | Protein: 0g | Carbohydrates: 8g | Fat: 0g | Fiber: 0g | Sugar: 7g

Anti-Inflammatory Smoothie

Prep Time: 10 minutes | Cooking Time: 0 minutes | Servings: 2

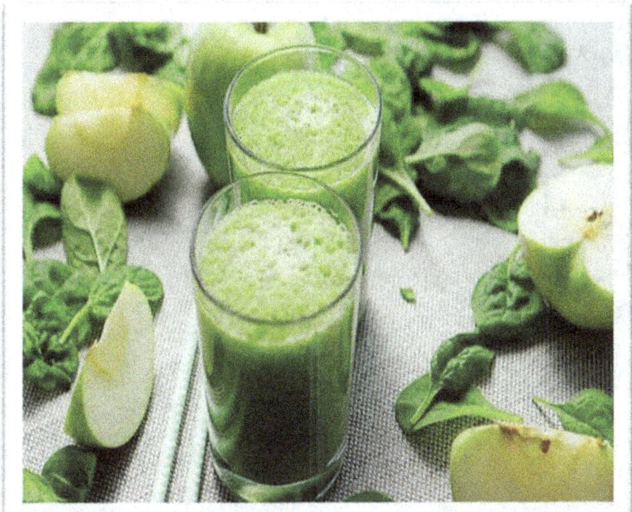

Ingredients:

- 1 cup frozen mango chunks
- 1 banana
- 1/2 cup unsweetened almond milk
- 1 teaspoon ground turmeric
- 1/2 teaspoon ground ginger
- 1/2 cup fresh spinach
- Toppings: sliced almonds, fresh berries, chia seeds

Instructions:

1. In a blender, combine mango, banana, almond milk, turmeric, ginger, and spinach. Blend until smooth.
2. Pour the smoothie into glass.
3. Top with sliced almonds, fresh berries, and chia seeds.
4. Serve immediately.

Nutritional Information: Calories: 180 | Protein: 3g | Carbohydrates: 40g | Fat: 3g | Fiber: 7g | Sugar: 25g

Refreshing Cucumber Lemonade

Prep Time: 10 minutes | Cooking Time: 0 minutes | Servings: 4

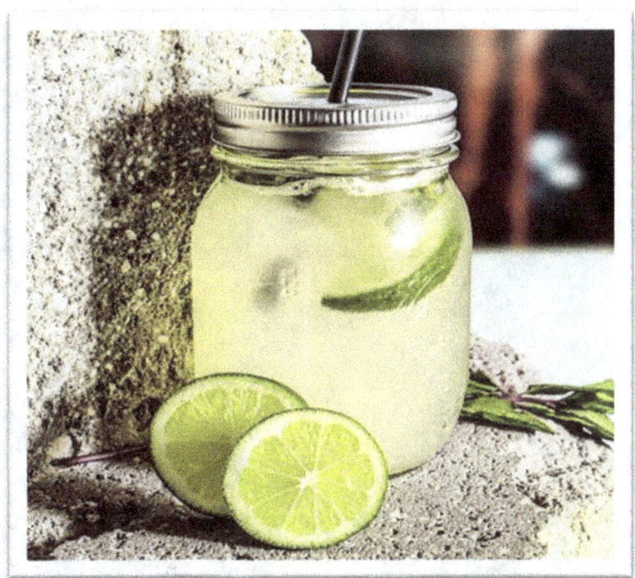

Ingredients:

- 1 cucumber, peeled and sliced
- Juice of 4 lemons
- 4 cups water
- 2 tablespoons honey
- Ice cubes
- Fresh mint leaves for garnish

Instructions:

1. In a blender, combine cucumber slices, lemon juice, water, and honey. Blend until smooth.
2. Strain the mixture through a fine mesh sieve into a pitcher.
3. Add ice cubes and stir to combine.
4. Garnish with fresh mint leaves.
5. Serve immediately.

Nutritional Information: Calories: 35 | Protein: 0g | Carbohydrates: 9g | Fat: 0g | Fiber: 0g | Sugar: 8g

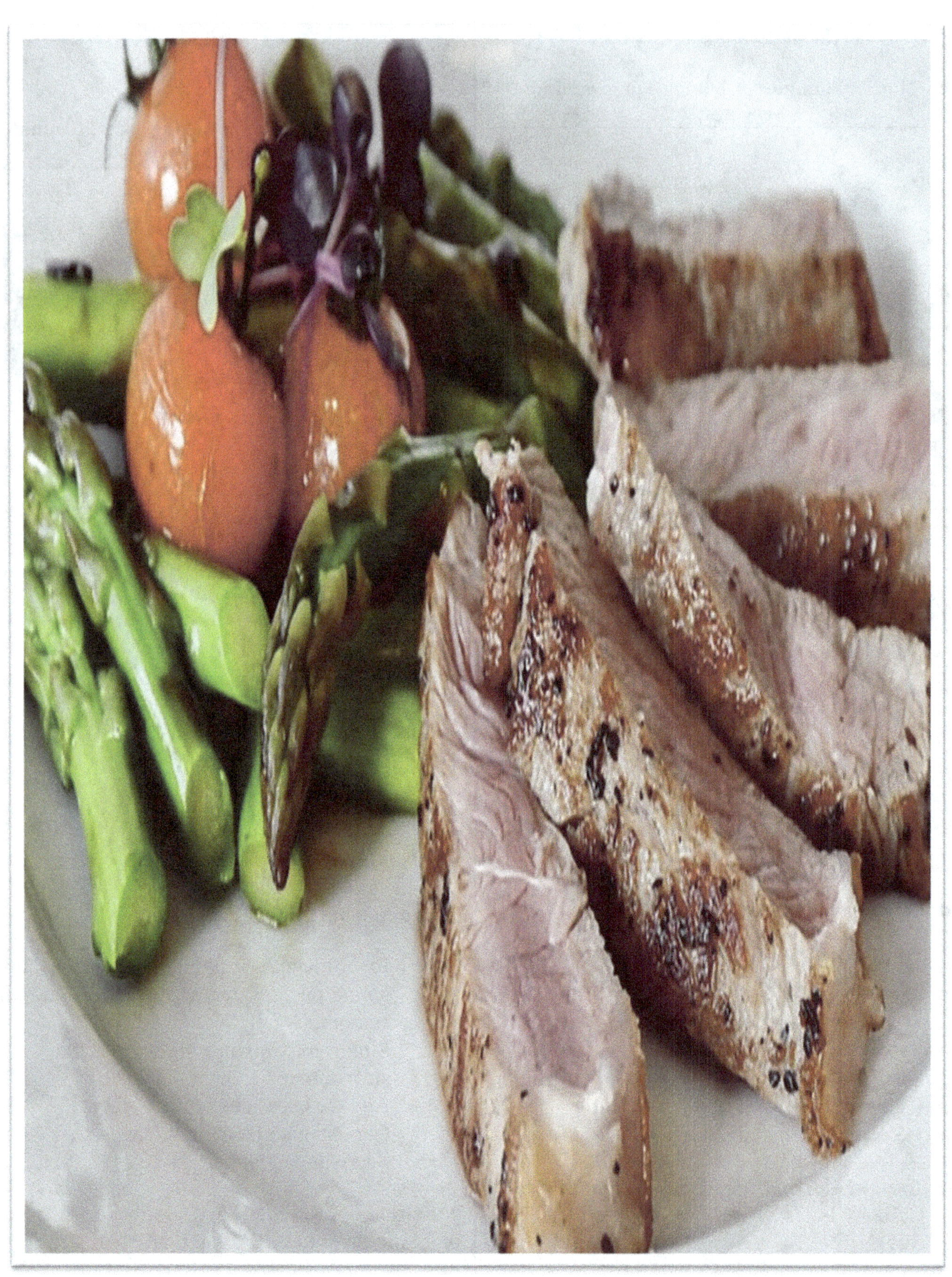

Turmeric Tahini Dressing

Prep Time: 5 minutes | Cooking Time: 0 minutes | Servings: 4

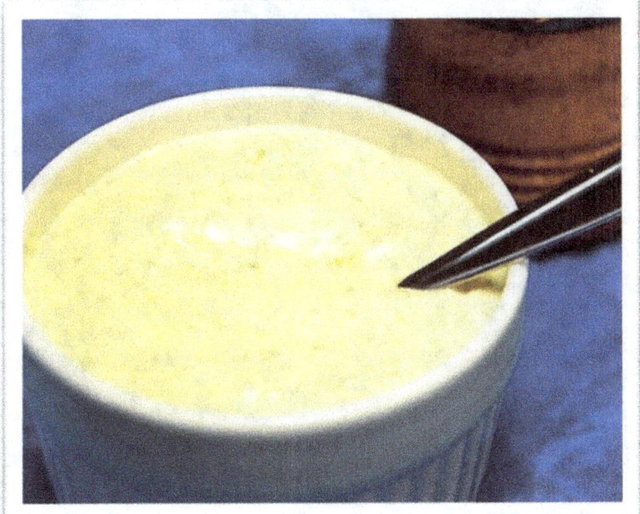

Ingredients:

- 1/4 cup tahini
- 1/4 cup water
- 1 tablespoon lemon juice
- 1 teaspoon ground turmeric
- 1 clove garlic, minced
- 1 tablespoon olive oil
- Salt and pepper to taste

Instructions:

1. In a small bowl, whisk together tahini, water, lemon juice, turmeric, garlic, olive oil, salt, and pepper until smooth.
2. Adjust the consistency with additional water if needed.
3. Serve immediately or refrigerate until ready to use.

Nutritional Information: Calories: 100 | Protein: 3g | Carbohydrates: 4g | Fat: 9g | Fiber: 2g | Sugar: 0g

Lemon Ginger Vinaigrette

Prep Time: 5 minutes | Cooking Time: 0 minutes | Servings: 4

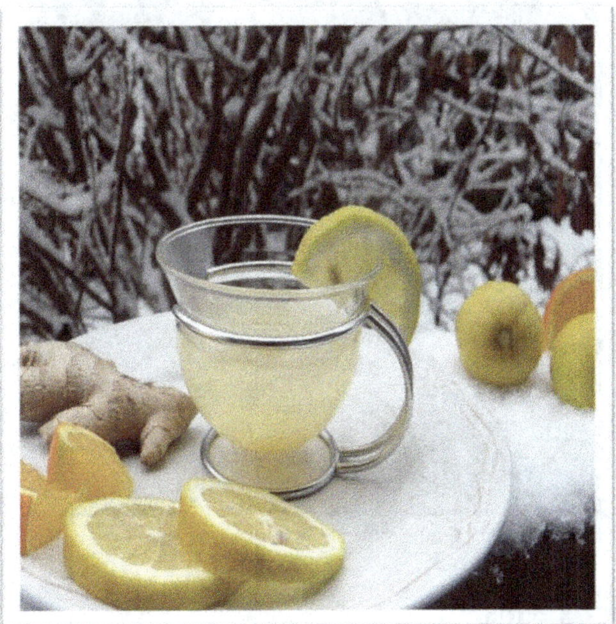

Ingredients:

- 1/4 cup olive oil
- 2 tablespoons lemon juice
- 1 tablespoon apple cider vinegar
- 1 teaspoon grated fresh ginger
- 1 teaspoon honey
- Salt and pepper to taste

Instructions:

1. In a small bowl, whisk together olive oil, lemon juice, apple cider vinegar, grated ginger, honey, salt, and pepper until well combined.
2. Serve immediately or refrigerate until ready to use.

Nutritional Information: Calories: 120 | Protein: 0g | Carbohydrates: 2g | Fat: 13g | Fiber: 0g | Sugar: 1g

Avocado Cilantro Dressing

Prep Time: 10 minutes | Cooking Time: 0 minutes | Servings: 4

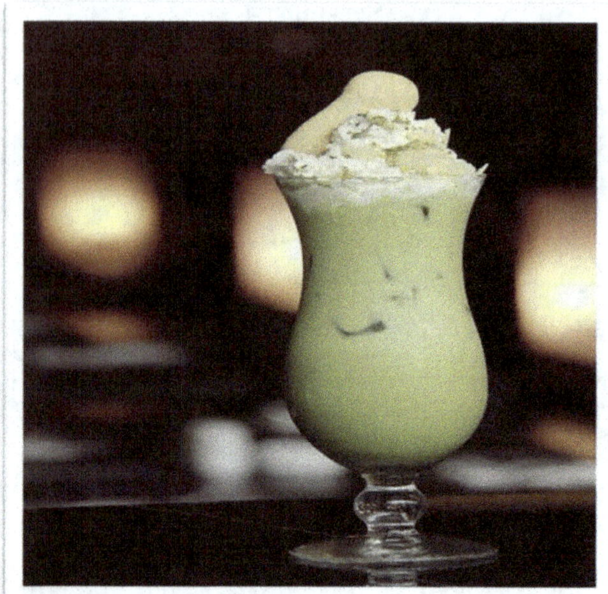

Ingredients:

- 1 ripe avocado
- 1/4 cup fresh cilantro leaves
- 1/4 cup Greek yogurt (or dairy-free yogurt)
- 2 tablespoons lime juice
- 1 clove garlic
- Salt and pepper to taste
- Water, as needed for thinning

Instructions:

1. In a blender, combine avocado, cilantro, Greek yogurt, lime juice, garlic, salt, and pepper. Blend until smooth.
2. Add water as needed to achieve desired consistency.
3. Serve immediately or refrigerate until ready to use.

Nutritional Information: Calories: 90 | Protein: 2g | Carbohydrates: 7g | Fat: 7g | Fiber: 3g | Sugar: 1g

Anti-Inflammatory Pesto

Prep Time: 10 minutes | Cooking Time: 0 minutes | Servings: 4

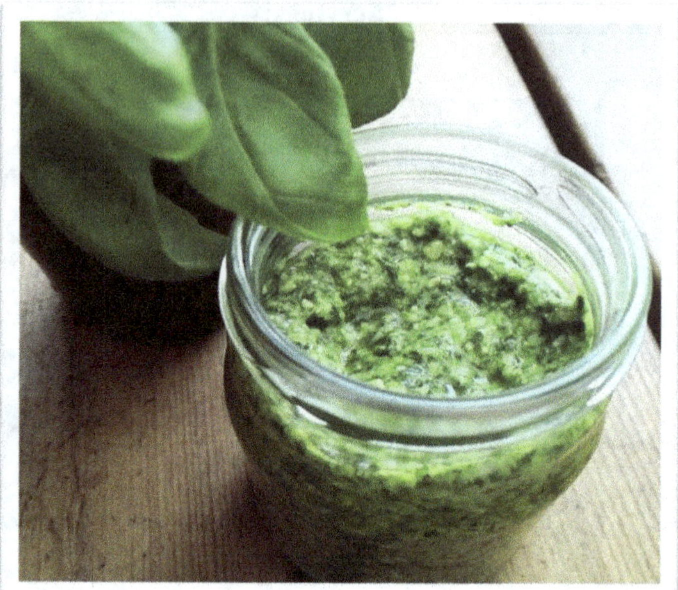

Ingredients:

- 2 cups fresh basil leaves
- 1/4 cup pine nuts
- 2 cloves garlic
- 1/4 cup olive oil
- 1/4 cup nutritional yeast (or Parmesan cheese)
- 1 teaspoon ground turmeric
- Salt and pepper to taste

Instructions:

1. In a food processor, combine basil leaves, pine nuts, garlic, olive oil, nutritional yeast, turmeric, salt, and pepper. Blend until smooth.
2. Adjust seasoning to taste.
3. Serve immediately or refrigerate until ready to use.

Nutritional Information: Calories: 130 | Protein: 3g | Carbohydrates: 3g | Fat: 13g | Fiber: 2g | Sugar: 0g

Spicy Almond Butter Sauce

Prep Time: 5 minutes | Cooking Time: 0 minutes | Servings: 4

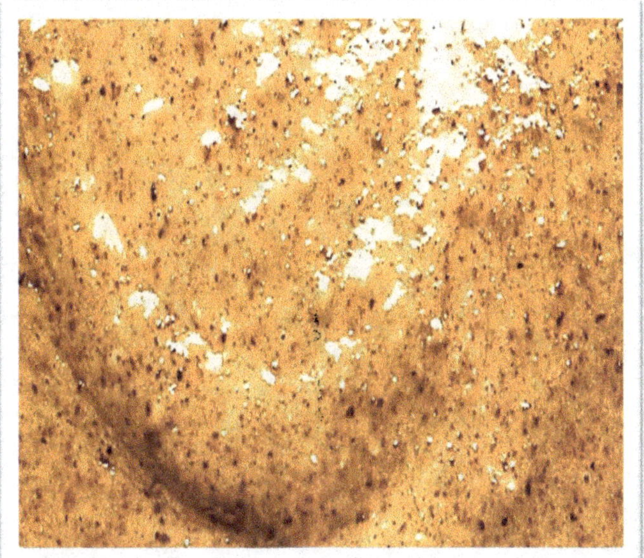

Ingredients:

- 1/4 cup almond butter
- 2 tablespoons soy sauce
- 1 tablespoon lime juice
- 1 tablespoon honey
- 1 clove garlic, minced
- 1/2 teaspoon red pepper flakes
- Water, as needed for thinning

Instructions:

1. In a small bowl, whisk together almond butter, soy sauce, lime juice, honey, garlic, and red pepper flakes until smooth.
2. Add water as needed to achieve desired consistency.
3. Serve immediately or refrigerate until ready to use.

Nutritional Information: Calories: 130 | Protein: 3g | Carbohydrates: 7g | Fat: 11g | Fiber: 2g | Sugar: 4g

Citrus Herb Dressing

Prep Time: 5 minutes | Cooking Time: 0 minutes | Servings: 4

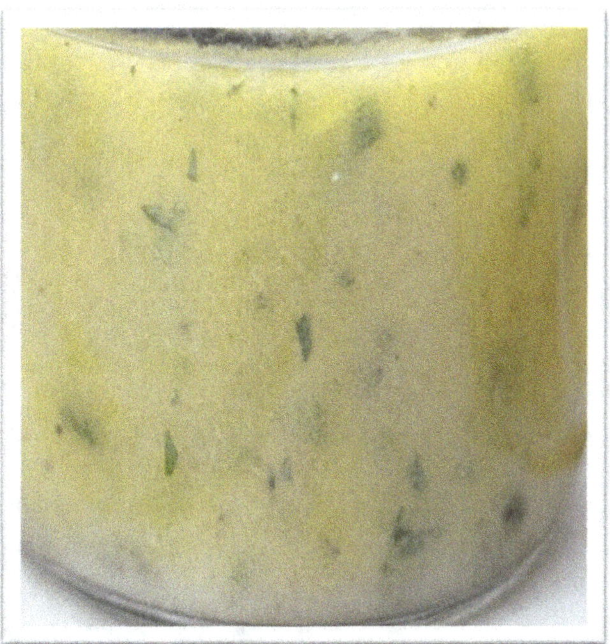

Ingredients:

- 1/4 cup olive oil
- 2 tablespoons orange juice
- 1 tablespoon lemon juice
- 1 tablespoon chopped fresh parsley
- 1 teaspoon Dijon mustard
- Salt and pepper to taste

Instructions:

1. In a small bowl, whisk together olive oil, orange juice, lemon juice, parsley, Dijon mustard, salt, and pepper until well combined.
2. Serve immediately or refrigerate until ready to use.

Nutritional Information: Calories: 120 | Protein: 0g | Carbohydrates: 2g | Fat: 13g | Fiber: 0g | Sugar: 1g

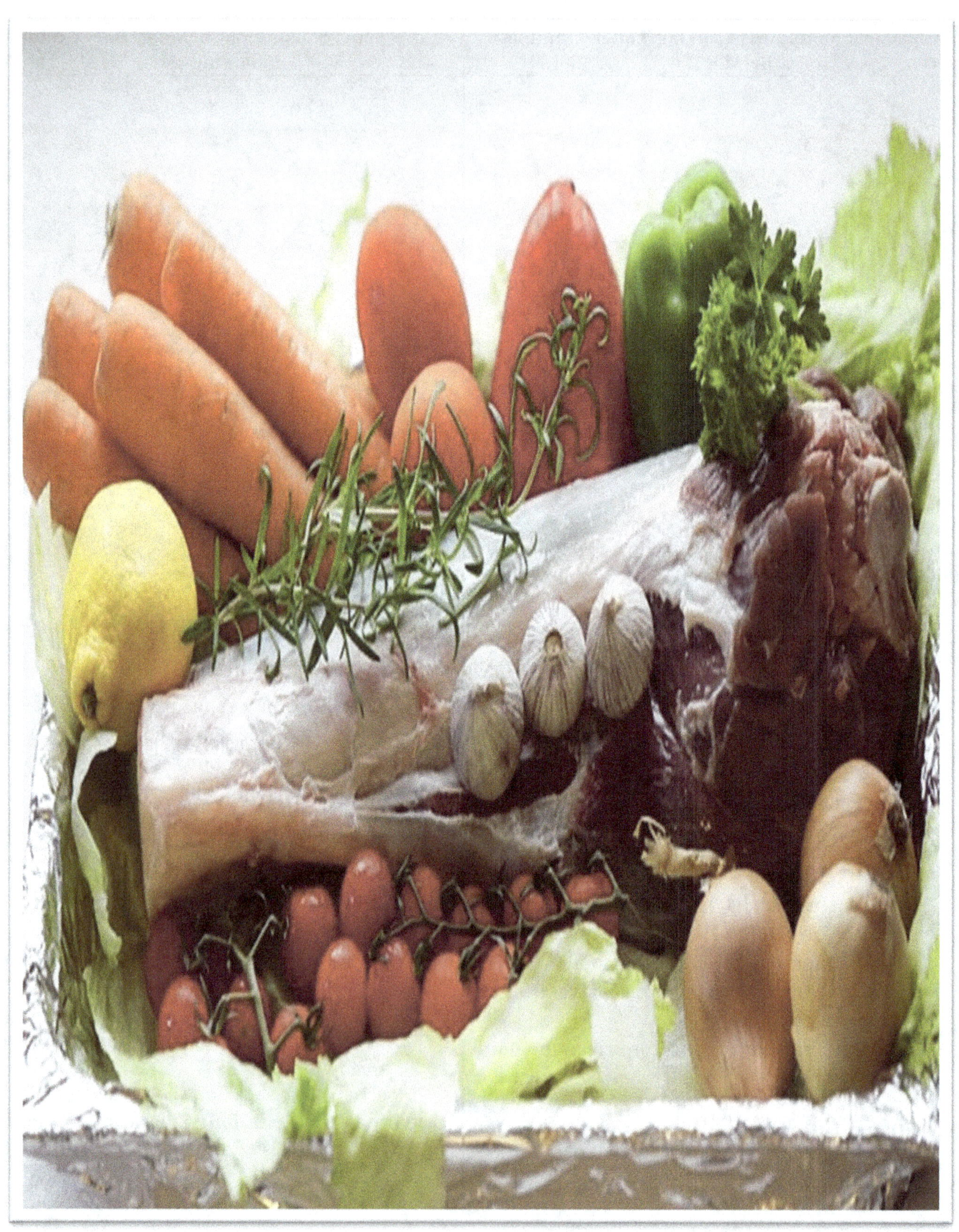

Many of us are trying to live healthier lives by exercising regularly and maintaining balanced diets. However, many of us still suffer from obesity, high blood pressure, type 2 diabetes, and high cholesterol, which increase the risk of conditions such as heart disease and stroke. The Complete Anti-Inflammatory Diet for Beginners is a diet to promote overall health and to reduce the risk of chronic diseases. This anti-inflammatory diet for beginners is about eating to avoid the metabolic conditions that lead to widespread inflammation, a major cause of heart disease, type 2 diabetes, arthritis, and several other chronic maladies. It is designed to help you improve your diet in light of the chronic inflammation that underlies these conditions. This diet is low-carb and low-fat which will enable you to help your body cleanse itself of the inflammation that is the common culprit of chronic disease. The anti-inflammatory diet is both flexible and provides a roadmap for more stringent adherence.

Allow this book to show you how making simple yet well-considered changes to your diet will lead to a happier, healthier future for you and your family. A host of recipes, guidelines, and tips for enjoying life in conjunction with the anti-inflammatory diet are included to help get you started. Even if you choose not to put yourself through the inconvenience of closely following the anti-inflammatory diet, understand that the health of our bodies cannot be achieved and possibly cannot even be pursued without the health of our immune system. The overall control and suppression of chronic inflammation will forever alter your diet and your recipe choices. Simply put, this book enables you to make well-informed food choices. With careful attention to both flavor and nutrition and gained mindfulness about inflammation, empowerment will be yours.

Tips for Maintaining an Anti-Inflammatory Diet

1. **Plan Your Meals**: Create a weekly diet plan that incorporates a range of foods that reduce inflammation. This helps ensure you get a balanced intake of nutrients and keeps your meals interesting.
2. **Prep in Advance**: Spend some time each week prepping ingredients like chopping vegetables, cooking grains, and marinating proteins. This makes meal preparation quicker and easier during busy days.
3. **Batch Cooking**: Cook larger portions of meals and store them in the refrigerator or freezer. This is particularly useful for soups, stews, and grain dishes that reheat well.
4. **Keep Healthy Snacks Handy**: Stock your pantry with healthy snacks like nuts, seeds, dried fruits, and cut-up vegetables. Having these ready-to-eat options can help you avoid reaching for inflammatory foods.
5. **Stay Hydrated**: Drink plenty of water throughout the day. You can also include herbal teas and infused water for variety.
6. **Experiment with Recipes**: Keep your diet exciting by trying new recipes and ingredients. This will help you discover new favorite dishes and avoid boredom.
7. **Listen to Your Body**: Observe how your body reacts to various foods. Everyone is unique, and some foods that are generally anti-inflammatory might not work well for you.
8. **Moderation is Key**: While it's important to focus on anti-inflammatory foods, it's also okay to indulge occasionally. Balance and moderation are essential for long-term sustainability.

Shopping List for Anti-Inflammatory Ingredients

Fruits and Vegetables:

- Berries (blueberries, strawberries, raspberries)
- Leafy greens (spinach, kale, Swiss chard)
- Cruciferous vegetables (broccoli, cauliflower, Brussels sprouts)
- Root vegetables (sweet potatoes, carrots, beets)
- Avocados
- Tomatoes
- Bell peppers

Healthy Fats:

- Olive oil
- Coconut oil
- Avocados
- Nuts (almonds, walnuts, cashews)
- Seeds (chia seeds, flaxseeds, hemp seeds)

Whole Grains:

- Quinoa
- Brown rice
- Oats
- Whole wheat products

Lean Proteins:

- Chicken
- Turkey
- Fish (salmon, mackerel, sardines)
- Tofu
- Tempeh
- Legumes (beans, lentils, chickpeas)

Herbs and Spices:

- Turmeric
- Ginger
- Garlic
- Cinnamon
- Black pepper
- Fresh herbs (basil, parsley, cilantro, mint)

Beverages:

- Green tea
- Herbal teas
- Coconut water

Other Essentials:

- Greek yogurt (or dairy-free yogurt)
- Apple cider vinegar
- Honey or maple syrup
- Tahini
- Nutritional yeast

30-DAY ANTI-INFLAMMATORY MEAL PLAN

Day	Breakfast	Lunch	Dinner	Snack
1	Turmeric and Ginger Smoothie	Mediterranean Quinoa Salad	Baked Salmon with Lemon and Dill	Hummus and Veggie Platter
2	Overnight Oats with Chia Seeds	Spinach and Strawberry Salad with Walnuts	Quinoa Stuffed Bell Peppers	Turmeric Roasted Chickpeas
3	Anti-Inflammatory Green Juice	Chickpea and Avocado Salad	Turmeric Chicken and Rice	Cucumber and Avocado Bites
4	Quinoa Breakfast Bowl with Berries	Kale and Blueberry Superfood Salad	Lentil and Vegetable Stir-Fry	Spicy Kale Chips
5	Avocado and Spinach Smoothie	Roasted Beet and Arugula Salad	Spaghetti Squash with Tomato and Basil	Almond and Berry Energy Balls
6	Sweet Potato and Black Bean Hash	Warm Lentil Salad with Lemon	Grilled Tofu with Ginger Soy Marinade	Fresh Vegetable Spring Rolls
7	Chia Seed Pudding with Berries	Cucumber, Tomato, and Feta Salad	Herb-Crusted Cod	Baked Zucchini Fries
8	Spinach and Mushroom Frittata	Mediterranean Quinoa Salad	Zucchini Noodles with Pesto	Roasted Red Pepper Hummus
9	Turmeric and Ginger Smoothie	Spinach and Strawberry Salad with Walnuts	Mushroom and Spinach Stuffed Portobellos	Hummus and Veggie Platter
10	Overnight Oats with Chia Seeds	Chickpea and Avocado Salad	Chickpea and Spinach Curry	Turmeric Roasted Chickpeas
11	Anti-Inflammatory Green Juice	Kale and Blueberry Superfood Salad	Roasted Cauliflower Steaks	Cucumber and Avocado Bites
12	Quinoa Breakfast Bowl with Berries	Roasted Beet and Arugula Salad	Baked Cod with Tomato and Olives	Spicy Kale Chips
13	Avocado and Spinach Smoothie	Warm Lentil Salad with Lemon	Sweet Potato and Black Bean Enchiladas	Almond and Berry Energy Balls
14	Sweet Potato and Black Bean Hash	Cucumber, Tomato, and Feta Salad	Vegan Lentil Loaf	Fresh Vegetable Spring Rolls
15	Chia Seed Pudding with Berries	Mediterranean Quinoa Salad	Chickpea and Sweet Potato Buddha Bowl	Baked Zucchini Fries

Day	Breakfast	Lunch	Dinner	Snack
16	Spinach and Mushroom Frittata	Spinach and Strawberry Salad with Walnuts	Cauliflower Tacos with Avocado Lime Sauce	Roasted Red Pepper Hummus
17	Turmeric and Ginger Smoothie	Chickpea and Avocado Salad	Eggplant and Chickpea Stew	Hummus and Veggie Platter
18	Overnight Oats with Chia Seeds	Kale and Blueberry Superfood Salad	Vegan Stuffed Peppers	Turmeric Roasted Chickpeas
19	Anti-Inflammatory Green Juice	Roasted Beet and Arugula Salad	Black Bean and Quinoa Salad	Cucumber and Avocado Bites
20	Quinoa Breakfast Bowl with Berries	Warm Lentil Salad with Lemon	Sweet Potato and Lentil Shepherd's Pie	Spicy Kale Chips
21	Avocado and Spinach Smoothie	Cucumber, Tomato, and Feta Salad	Vegan Mushroom Stroganoff	Almond and Berry Energy Balls
22	Sweet Potato and Black Bean Hash	Mediterranean Quinoa Salad	Baked Salmon with Lemon and Dill	Fresh Vegetable Spring Rolls
23	Chia Seed Pudding with Berries	Spinach and Strawberry Salad with Walnuts	Quinoa Stuffed Bell Peppers	Baked Zucchini Fries
24	Spinach and Mushroom Frittata	Chickpea and Avocado Salad	Turmeric Chicken and Rice	Roasted Red Pepper Hummus
25	Turmeric and Ginger Smoothie	Kale and Blueberry Superfood Salad	Lentil and Vegetable Stir-Fry	Hummus and Veggie Platter
26	Overnight Oats with Chia Seeds	Roasted Beet and Arugula Salad	Spaghetti Squash with Tomato and Basil	Turmeric Roasted Chickpeas
27	Anti-Inflammatory Green Juice	Warm Lentil Salad with Lemon	Grilled Tofu with Ginger Soy Marinade	Cucumber and Avocado Bites
28	Quinoa Breakfast Bowl with Berries	Cucumber, Tomato, and Feta Salad	Herb-Crusted Cod	Spicy Kale Chips
29	Avocado and Spinach Smoothie	Mediterranean Quinoa Salad	Zucchini Noodles with Pesto	Almond and Berry Energy Balls
30	Sweet Potato and Black Bean Hash	Spinach and Strawberry Salad with Walnuts	Mushroom and Spinach Stuffed Portobellos	Fresh Vegetable Spring Rolls

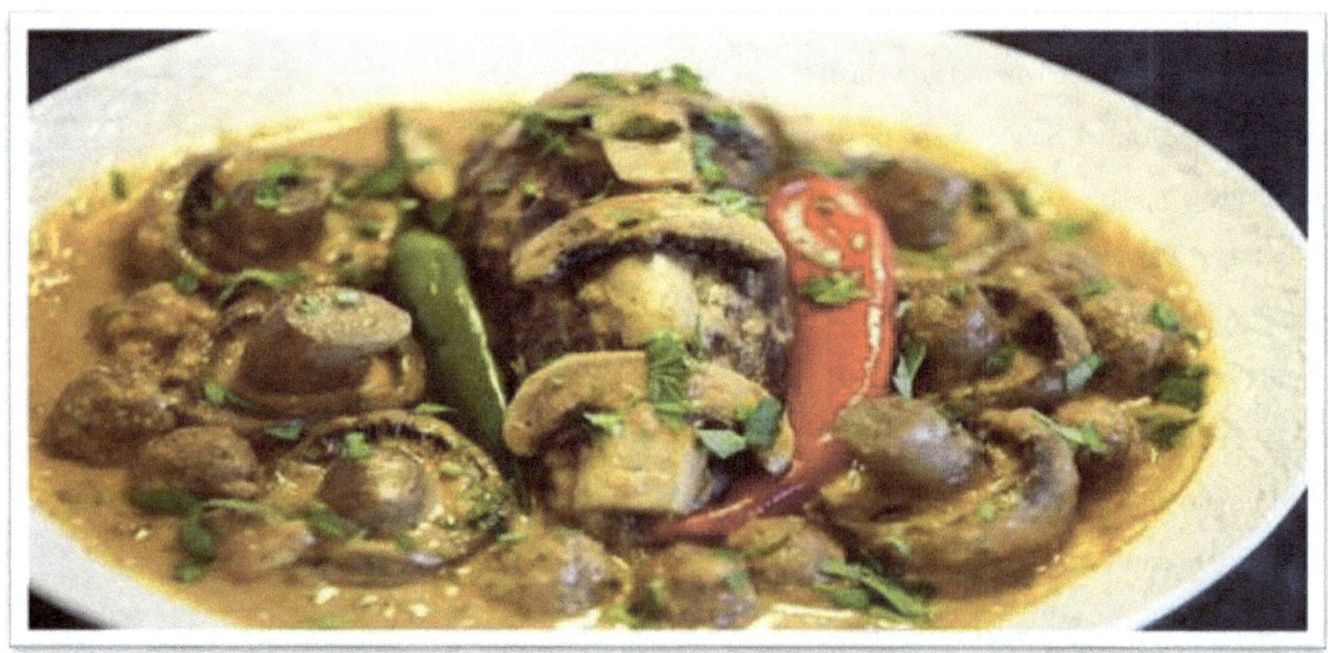

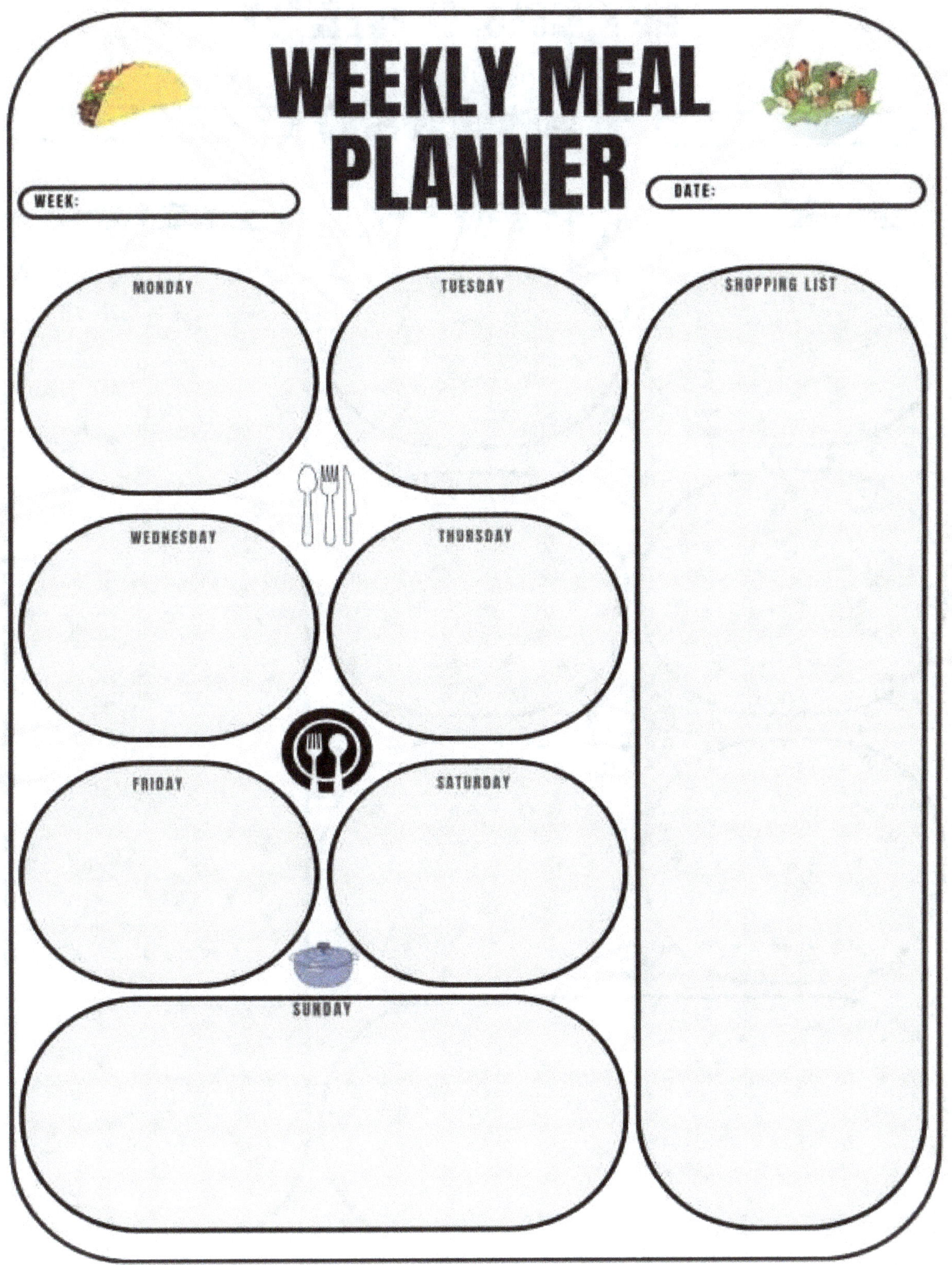

WEEKLY MEAL PLANNER
WEEK:
DATE:
MONDAY
TUESDAY
SHOPPING LIST
WEDNESDAY
THURSDAY
FRIDAY
SATURDAY
SUNDAY

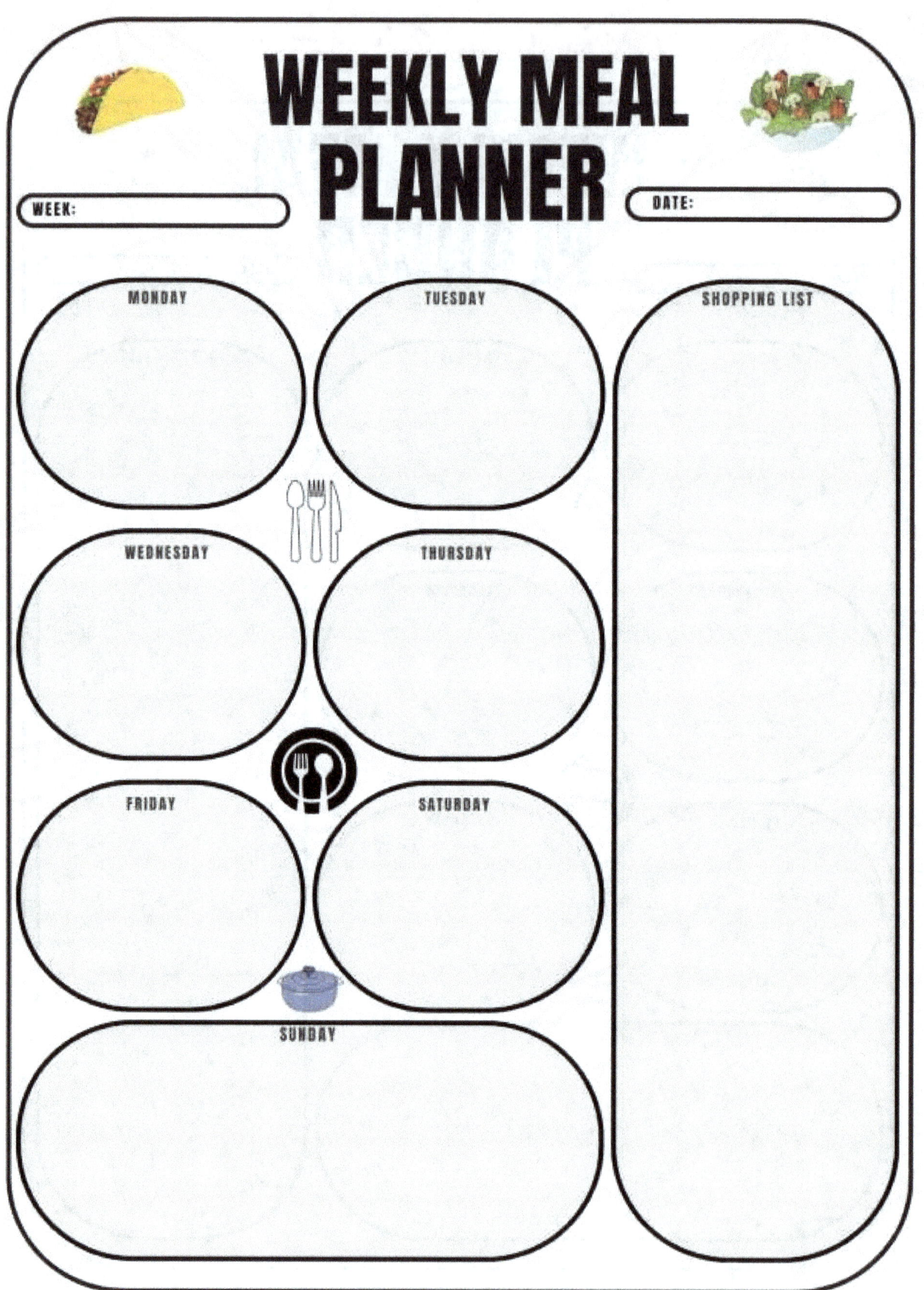
WEEKLY MEAL PLANNER
WEEK:
DATE:
MONDAY
TUESDAY
SHOPPING LIST
WEDNESDAY
THURSDAY
FRIDAY
SATURDAY
SUNDAY

WEEKLY MEAL PLANNER

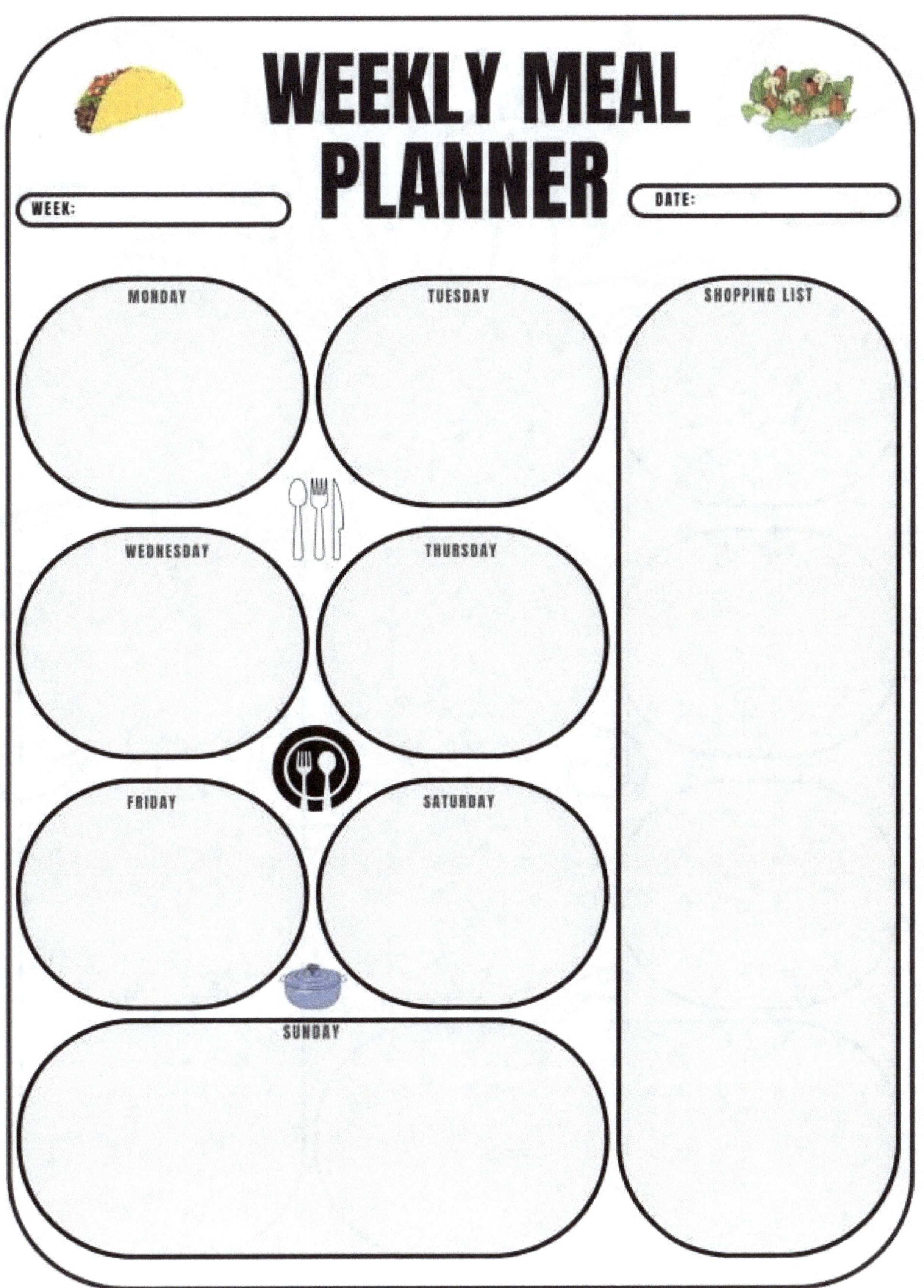

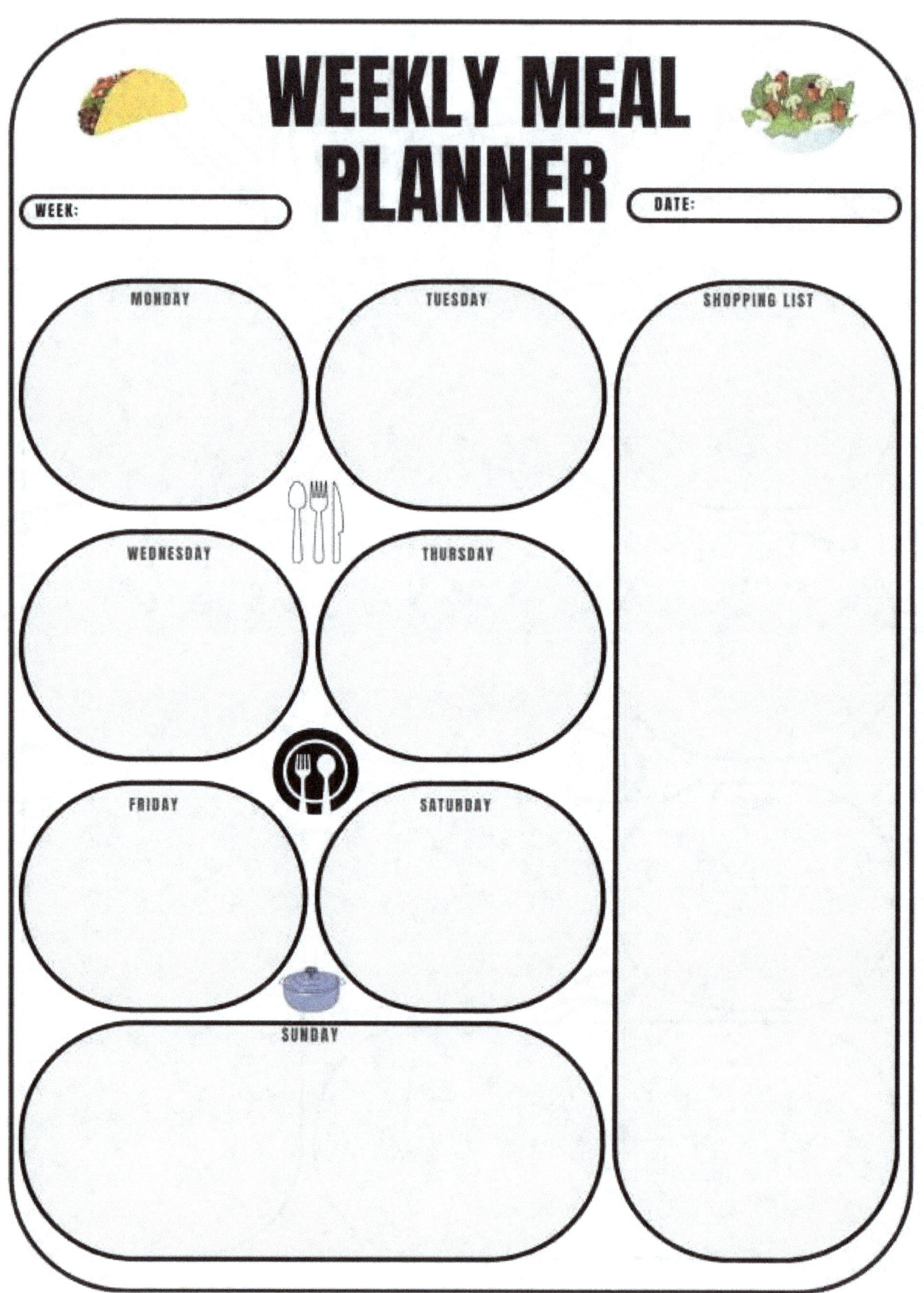
WEEKLY MEAL PLANNER
WEEK:
DATE:
MONDAY
TUESDAY
SHOPPING LIST
WEDNESDAY
THURSDAY
FRIDAY
SATURDAY
SUNDAY

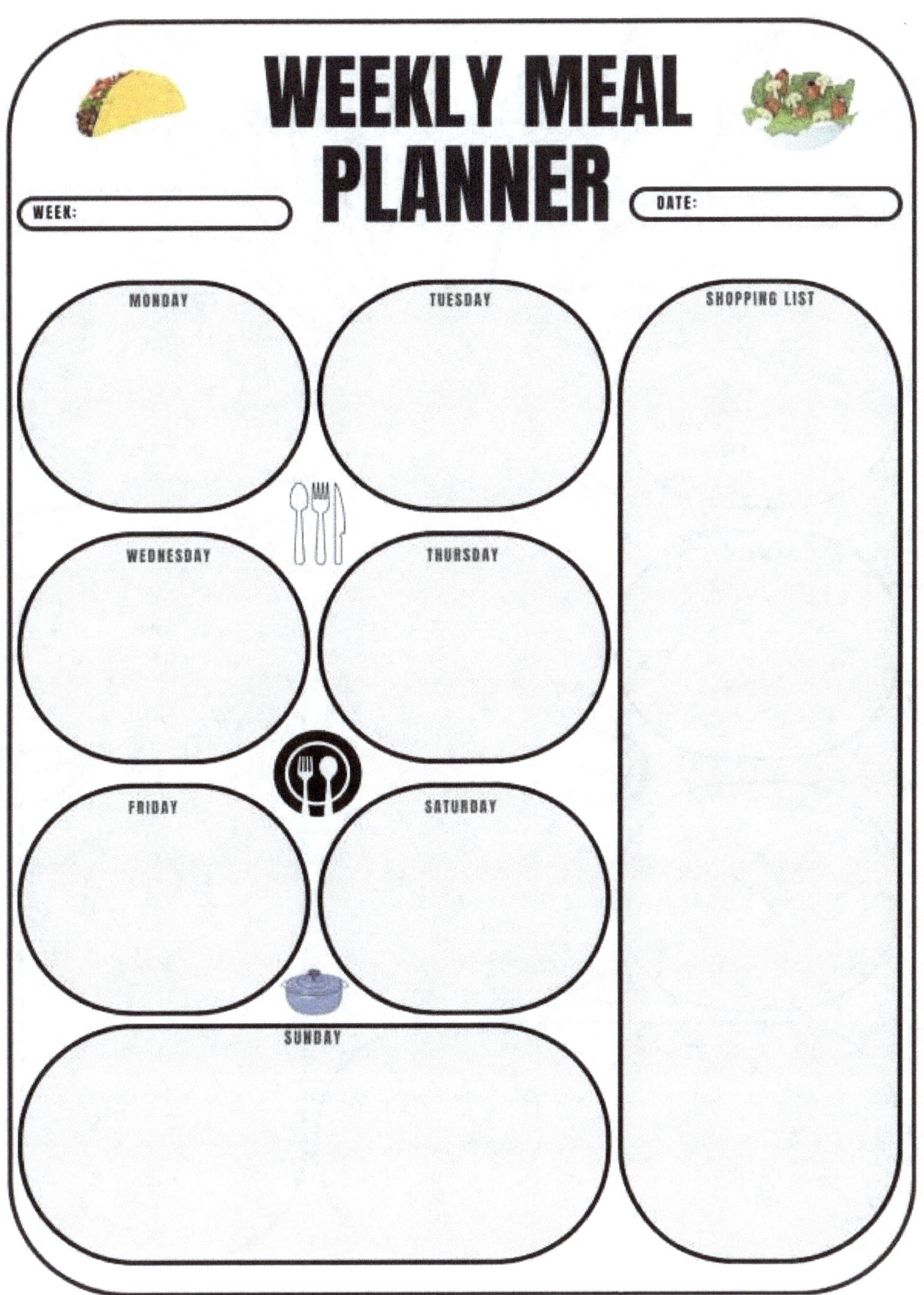

WEEKLY MEAL PLANNER
WEEK:
DATE:
MONDAY
TUESDAY
SHOPPING LIST
WEDNESDAY
THURSDAY
FRIDAY
SATURDAY
SUNDAY

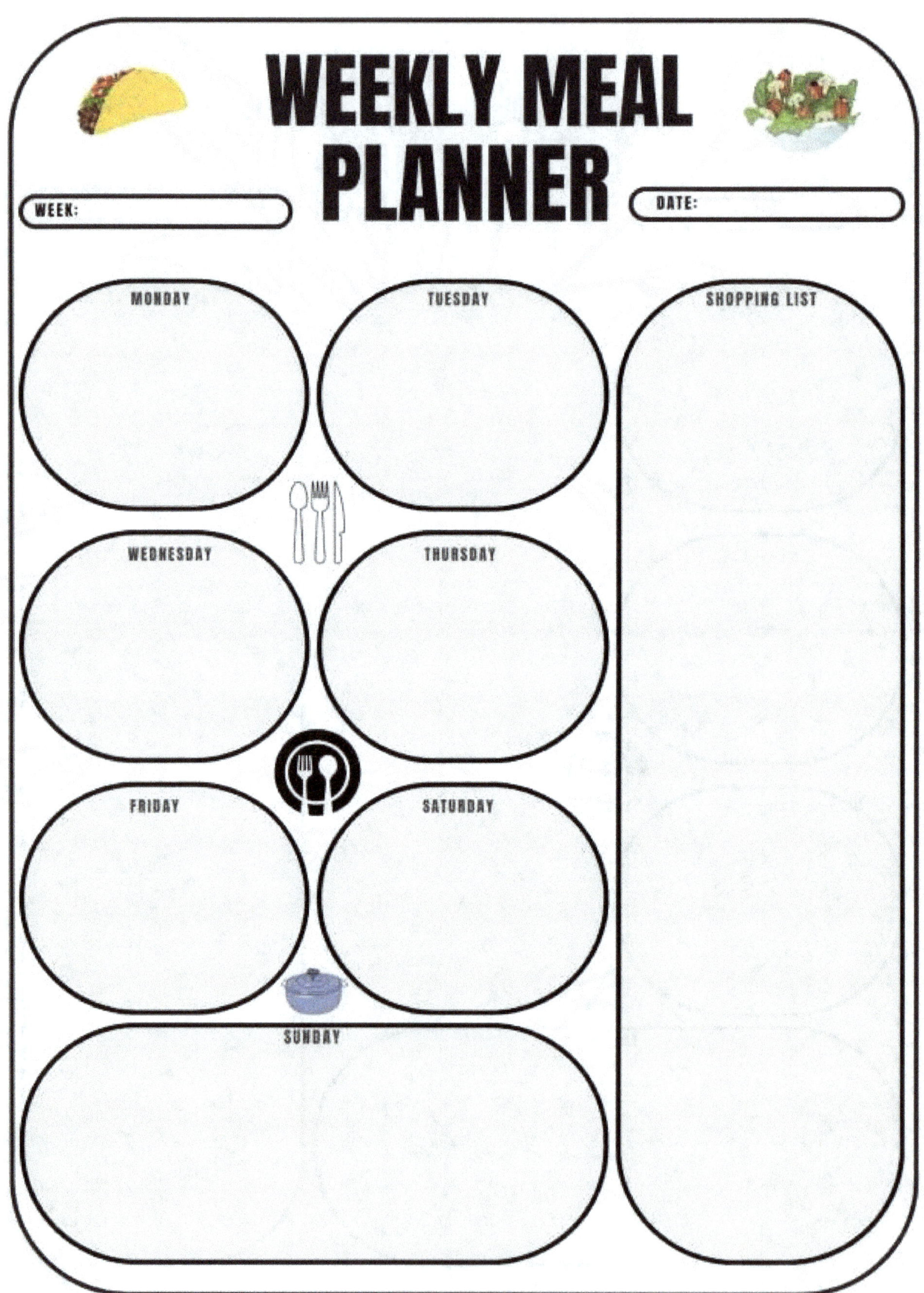

WEEKLY MEAL PLANNER
WEEK:
DATE:
MONDAY
TUESDAY
SHOPPING LIST
WEDNESDAY
THURSDAY
FRIDAY
SATURDAY
SUNDAY

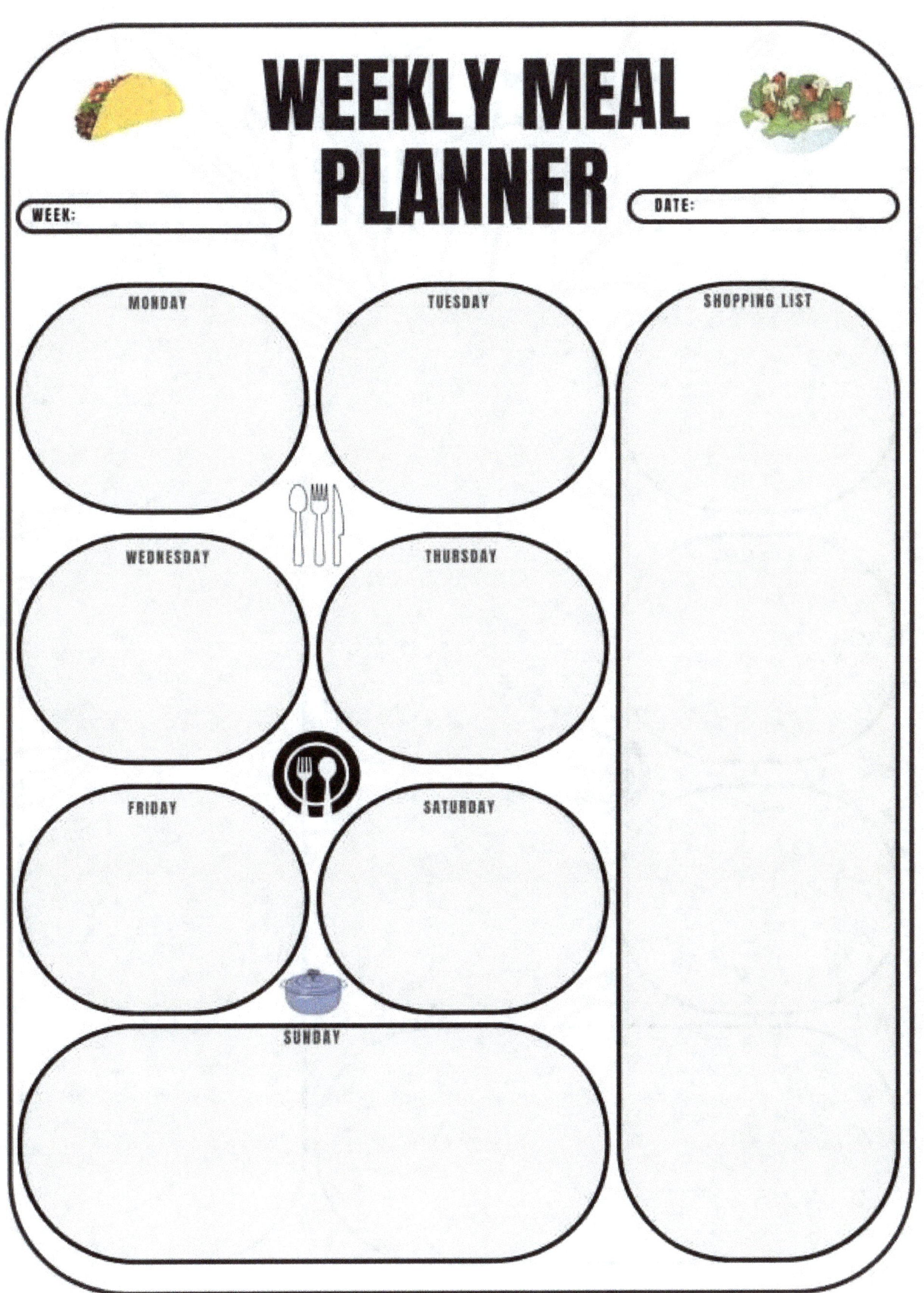

WEEKLY MEAL PLANNER
WEEK:
DATE:
MONDAY
TUESDAY
SHOPPING LIST
WEDNESDAY
THURSDAY
FRIDAY
SATURDAY
SUNDAY

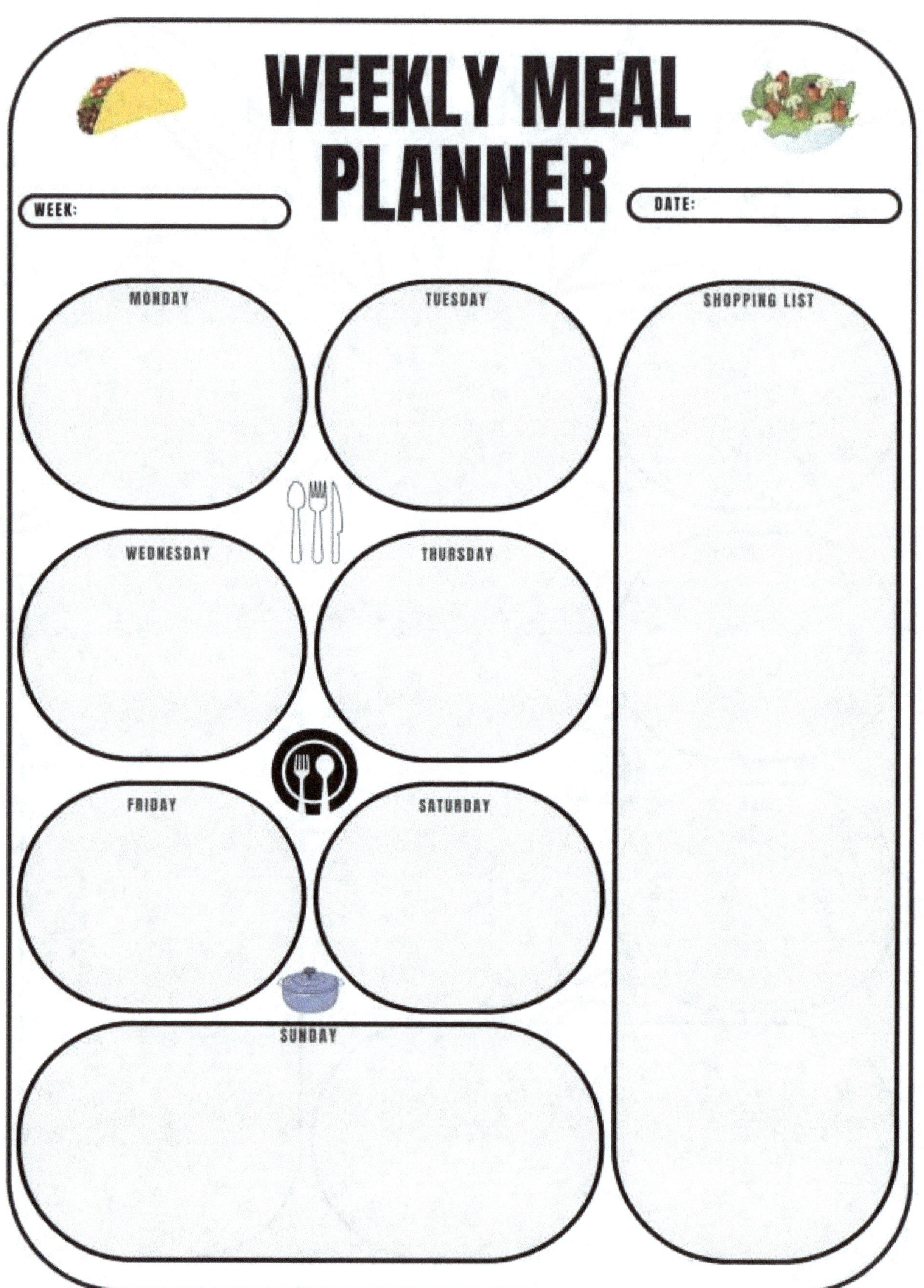

WEEKLY MEAL PLANNER
WEEK:
DATE:
MONDAY
TUESDAY
SHOPPING LIST
WEDNESDAY
THURSDAY
FRIDAY
SATURDAY
SUNDAY

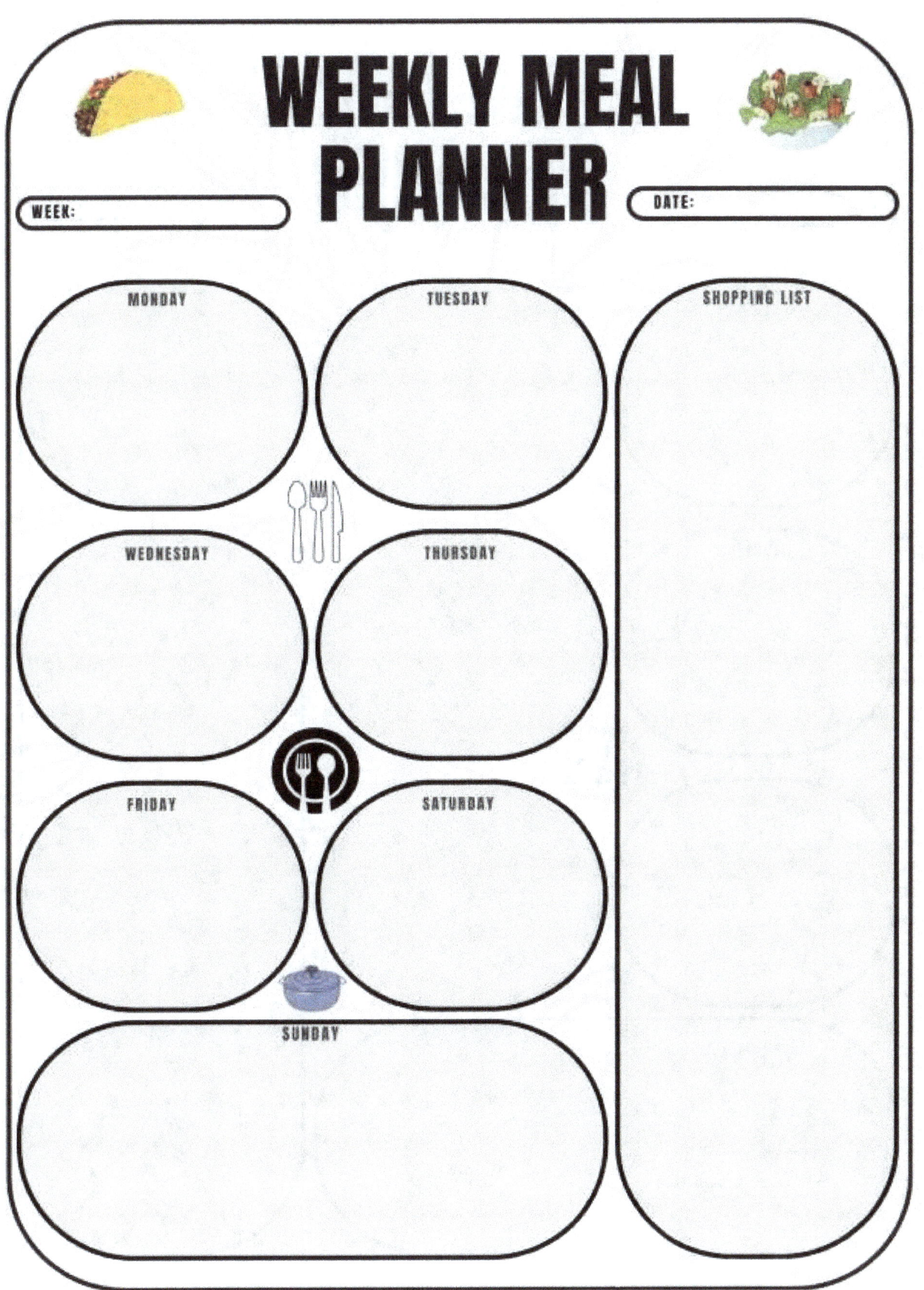

WEEKLY MEAL PLANNER
WEEK:
DATE:
MONDAY
TUESDAY
SHOPPING LIST
WEDNESDAY
THURSDAY
FRIDAY
SATURDAY
SUNDAY

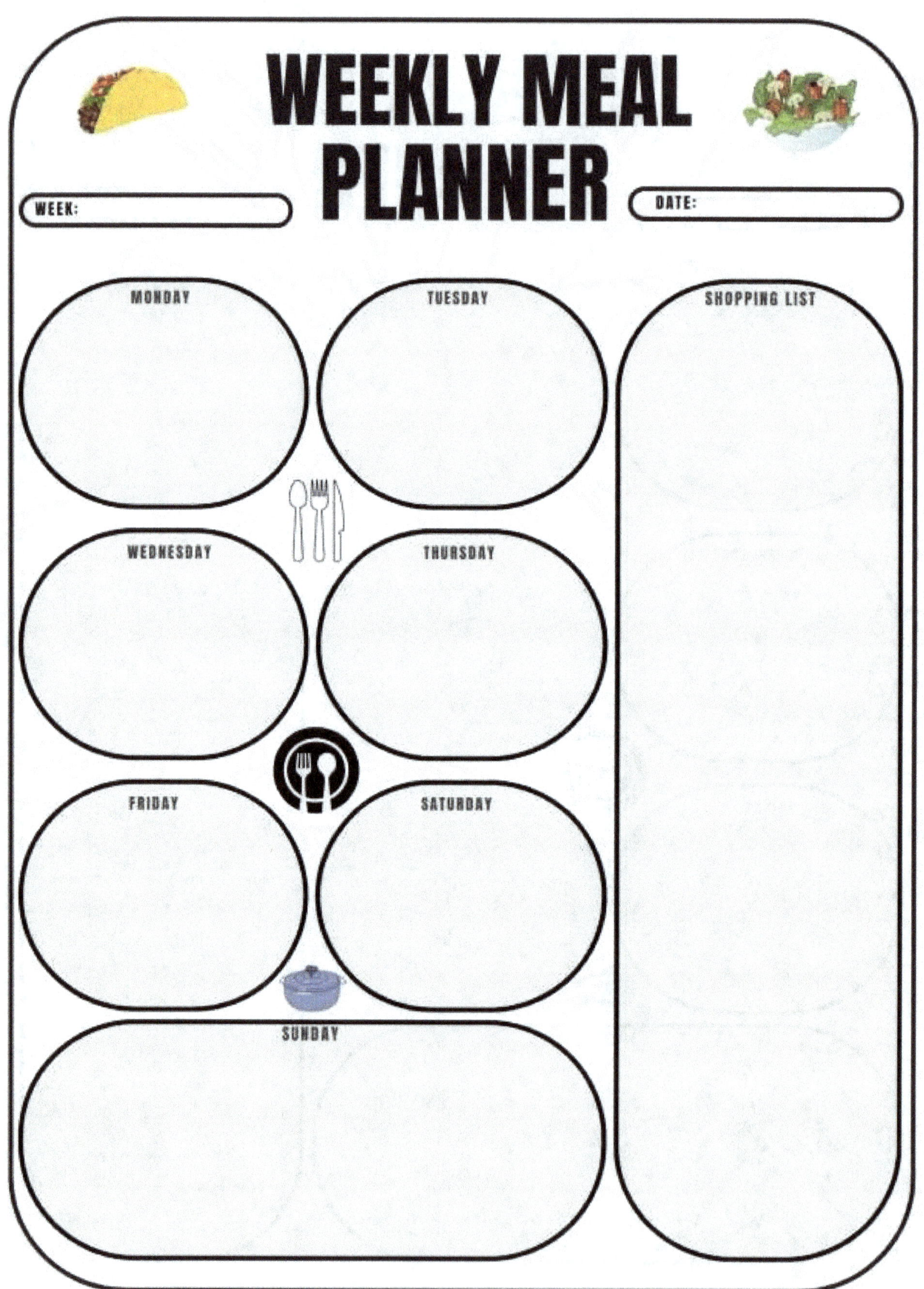
WEEKLY MEAL PLANNER
WEEK:
DATE:
MONDAY
TUESDAY
SHOPPING LIST
WEDNESDAY
THURSDAY
FRIDAY
SATURDAY
SUNDAY